Integra

Integrated Clinical Science

Other titles:

Cardiovascular Disease
Professor JR Hampton

Psychiatry
Professor JL Gibbons

Nephro-urology
Professor AW Asscher
Professor DB Moffat

Respiratory Disease
GM Sterling

Musculoskeletal Disease
Professor V Wright
Professor R Dickson

Gastroenterology
P Jones, P Brunt,
NAG Mowat

Neurology
RW Ross Russell

Endocrinology
Professor CRW Edwards

Projected

Human Health and the Environment

Reproduction and Development

Integrated Clinical Science

Haematology

Edited by

John C. Cawley MD, PhD, MRCP, MRCPath

Reader in Haematology, and Honorary Consultant Physician,
University College Hospital, London

Series Editor

George P McNicol, MD, PhD, FRCP
(Lond, Edin, Glasg), FRCPath, Hon FACP

Principal and Vice Chancellor, University of Aberdeen. Lately Professor of
Medicine, The University of Leeds, and Head, The University Department
of Medicine, The General Infirmary, Leeds

William Heinemann Medical Books Ltd
London

ISBN 0-433-16601-0

© 1983 William Heinemann Medical Books Ltd,
   23 Bedford Square,
   London WC1B 3HH

First published 1983
Reprinted 1985

Printed and bound in Great Britain by the
Alden Press, Oxford

Contents

Preface

It is clearly desirable on educational grounds to adopt and teach a rational approach to the management of patients, whereby the basic scientific knowledge, the applied science and the art of clinical practice are brought together in an integrated way. Progress has been made in this direction, but after twenty-five years of good intentions, teaching in many medical schools is still split up into three large compartments, preclinical, paraclinical and clinical, and further subdivided on a disciplinary basis. Lip-service is paid to integration, but what emerges is often at best a coordinated rather than an integrated curriculum. Publication of the INTE-GRATED CLINICAL SCIENCE series reflects the need felt in many quarters for a truly integrated textbook series, and is also intended as a stimulus to further reform of the curriculum.

The complete series will cover the core of clinical teaching, each volume dealing with a particular body system. Revision material in the basic sciences of anatomy, physiology, biochemistry and pharmacology is presented at the level of detail appropriate for Final MB examinations, and subsequently for rational clinical practice. Integration between the volumes ensures complete and consistent coverage of these areas, and similar principles govern the treatment of the clinical disciplines of medicine, surgery, pathology, micro-biology, immunology and epidemiology.

The series is planned to give a reasoned rather than a purely descriptive account of clinical practice and its scientific basis.

Clinical manifestations are described in relation to the disorders of structure and function which occur in a disease process. Illustrations are used extensively, and are an integral part of the text.

The editors for each volume, well-known as authorities and teachers in their fields, have been recruited from medical schools throughout the UK. Chapter contributors are even more widely distributed, and coordination between the volumes has been super-vised by a distinguished team of specialists.

Each volume in the series represents a component in an overall plan of approach to clinical teaching. It is intended, nevertheless, that every volume should be self-sufficient as an account of its own subject area, and all the basic and clinical science with which an undergraduate could reasonably be expected to be familiar is presented in the appropriate volume. It is expected that, whether studied individually or as a series, the volumes of INTEGRATED CLINICAL SCIENCE will meet a major need, assisting teachers and students to adopt a more rational and holistic approach in learning to care for the sick.

George P McNicol
Series Editor

Contributors

JC Cawley
Reader and Honorary Consultant
Department of Haematology
University College
London

JM England
Consultant Haematologist
Watford General Hospital
and Honorary Senior Lecturer and Consultant
St Mary's Hospital Medical School
London

CD Forbes
Senior Lecturer and Honorary Consultant
  Physician
University Department of Medicine
Royal Infirmary
Glasgow

ST Holgate
Senior Lecturer and Honorary Consultant
Department of Medicine
Southampton General Hospital

GDO Lowe
Lecturer in Medicine
University Department of Medicine
Royal Infirmary
Glasgow

KG Patterson
Consultant Haematologist
Barking General Hospital
London

AH Waters
Professor and Honorary Consultant Haematologist
Department of Haematology
St Bartholomew's Hospital
London

Advisory Editors

Professor A Stuart Douglas
Department of Medicine, University of Aberdeen

Pathology: Professor CC Bird
            Institute of Pathology
            University of Leeds

Physiology: Professor PH Fentem
            Department of Physiology and
                Pharmacology
            Nottingham University

Biochemistry: Dr RM Denton
            Reader in Biochemistry
            University of Bristol

Anatomy: Professor RL Holmes
            Department of Anatomy
            University of Leeds

Pharmacology: Professor AM Breckenridge
            Department of Clinical
                Pharmacology
            Liverpool University

Introduction

In accord with the general aim of the series to which it belongs, the purpose of this volume is to present, in an appropriate up-to-date scientific setting, the core material of haematology for the undergraduate student. The subject matter of haematology has been taken to include the lymphoreticular system as well as the blood and bone marrow. In addition, host defence has been included since this so intimately involves the haemopoietic and lymphoreticular systems.

The book consists of six chapters. Chapter 1 serves as an introduction and outlines the basic structure and function of the haemopoietic and lymphoreticular systems, dealing briefly with immunology and basic haematological investigations.

Chapter 2 considers the important anaemias from a mainly aetiological point of view, but at the same time gives the student an insight into classification based upon red-cell size.

Chapter 3 deals with blood transfusion in its broad sense and reflects the current importance of blood component therapy. The basic concepts of blood-transfusion serology are presented in a clinical context. The chapter includes a section on haemolytic disease of the newborn.

Chapters 4 and 5 deal with the related areas of haemostasis and thrombosis. While dealing with the established subjects of congenital coagulation disorders and clinical thrombosis, they give due emphasis to the platelet–vessel wall interactions so currently topical and relevant to degenerative vascular disease.

The volume concludes with a chapter on the main haematological malignancies, including the lymphomas.

It is intended that the volume should be to a large extent self-sufficient and not require continual reference to others in the series. Inevitably, therefore, there will be some overlap with other volumes.

Although core material is the prime concern of the volume, it is hoped that sufficient detail has been included to interest the more enterprising student and to provide a basis for further study in haematology.

The Haemopoietic and Lymphoreticular Systems

INTRODUCTION

The haematologist is concerned with disorders of the blood, and the blood-forming (haemopoietic) and lymphoreticular systems. The purpose of this introductory chapter is to outline the aspects of the structure and function of these closely related systems which are relevant to haematologists. One such function – host defence against infection – will be considered here in slightly greater detail since it is not considered elsewhere in the volume. The chapter concludes with a brief section on simple laboratory investigation to show how this can provide important information about the haemopoietic system.

BLOOD

When anticoagulated whole blood is allowed to settle, it reveals its three major components: red cells (erythrocytes); buffy coat consisting of white cells (leucocytes) and platelets; and plasma (Fig. 1.1).

Red Cells

Erythrocytes are biconcave discs with an average diameter of approximately 8 μ; their relative excess of surface over volume makes them very deformable and allows them to pass through the microcirculation, whose minimum diameter is considerably less than 8 μ.

Mature circulating erythrocytes possess a complex limiting membrane but lack nuclei and other subcellular organelles; their main contents are haemoglobin and a variety of enzymes and metabolic intermediates which are essential to the proper functioning of the haemoglobin and to maintaining the integrity of the cell.

Haemoglobin (Hb)

Haemoglobins are tetramers consisting of two α and two non-α globin chains, each with its own iron-containing haem group. The important normal haemoglobins are: HbA (the major adult haemoglobin) $\alpha_2\beta_2$; HbA$_2$

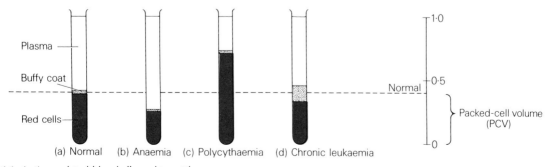

Fig. 1.1 *Anticoagulated blood allowed to settle.*

(a) Normal   (b) Anaemia   (c) Polycythaemia   (d) Chronic leukaemia

(the minor adult haemoglobin) $\alpha_2\delta_2$; and HbF (fetal haemoglobin) $\alpha_2\gamma_2$. During most of fetal life, HbF is predominant; at birth, HbA constitutes less than one-third of the Hb present. After birth, HbF formation rapidly declines so that, by one year, HbF makes up only 2–3% of the Hb; by five years, adult proportions are present (HbA > 95%; HbA$_2$ < 3.5%; HbF < 1.5%).

The primary function of Hb is oxygen transport, which is brought about by reversible binding of one molecule of oxygen (O_2) by each haem group. This reversible binding is accompanied by complex changes in the association of globin chains within the globin tetramer and, in the reduced state, with binding of the glycolytic intermediate, 2,3-diphosphoglycerate (2,3-DPG) (see below). This binding stabilises Hb in its deoxy configuration, thereby reducing its oxygen affinity. These complex cooperative interactions determine the physiologically advantageous pattern of uptake (in the lungs) and delivery (to the tissues) of oxygen reflected in the sigmoidal oxygen dissociation curve (Fig. 1.2). The steep part of the curve occurs around the partial pressure of oxygen (PO_2) found in the tissues, and this makes possible large changes in oxygen binding with only small changes in oxygen tension; in contrast, at the higher levels of PO_2 found in the lungs, substantial changes in O_2 tension have only a minor effect on the oxygen saturation of Hb. The effect of 2,3-DPG on oxygen dissociation has already been mentioned, but a number of other factors are also important (Fig. 1.2). Factors that shift the curve to the right increase the efficiency of O_2 delivery, while factors causing a left shift have the opposite effect. In addition, the oxygen dissociation curve is influenced by the structure of Hb itself. For example, the oxygen dissociation curve of HbF is shifted to the left and the molecule has a higher oxygen affinity than HbA. Mutations affecting areas at which α and β chains interact during O_2 binding, or at which 2,3-DPG binds to Hb, may produce high or low affinity haemoglobins, and these in turn may result in polycythaemia or anaemia respectively.

Red-cell metabolism

Erythrocyte metabolism is directed towards two main ends: the formation of ATP to provide the energy necessary for preserving the intracellular ionic environment, and the production of reducing power in the

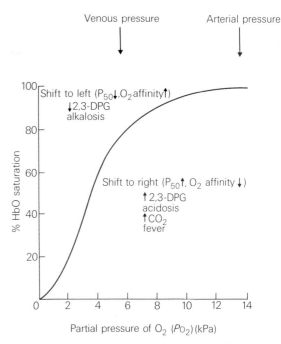

Fig. 1.2 *The oxygen dissociation curve. The effect of pH is termed the Bohr effect and accounts for enhanced O_2 delivery in the acid micro-environment of hypoxic tissues. At the usual venous oxygen tension ($\simeq$5.3 kPa) Hb is approximately 70% saturated. At normal arterial oxygen tension ($\simeq$13 kPa) Hb is completely saturated. NB: 1 mmHg = 0.133 kPa.*

form of NADH and NADPH to prevent oxidative damage to Hb and other intracellular constituents.

Glucose is the red cell's sole source of energy; approximately 90% is metabolised by anaerobic glycolysis (Embden–Meyerhof pathway), while about 10% is normally metabolised by the pentose phosphate pathway (hexose monophosphate shunt) (Fig. 1.3). Anaerobic glycolysis contributes ATP and NADH, while the pentose phosphate pathway produces NADPH which, via reduced glutathione, prevents oxidative damage to the sulphydryl groups of Hb and other cell constituents. In addition, a sidearm of glycolysis provides the 2,3-DPG important in the cell's adaptive mechanisms for changing oxygen affinity.

Breakdown of red cells

After formation (see p. 13) and release from the marrow, normal erythrocytes live for approximately 120 days before they are removed by the reticuloendothelial

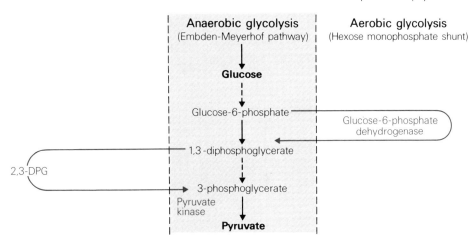

Fig. 1.3 *Simplified representation of red-cell metabolism. Many enzyme abnormalities of these pathways have been described, but the two most common enzymopathies are glucose-6-phosphate dehydrogenase and pyruvate kinase deficiencies, which are shown here. In pyruvate kinase deficiency, 2,3-DPG is increased; it is normal in glucose-6-phosphate dehydrogenase deficiency.*

system (see p. 15), mainly in the spleen. The precise mechanisms by which the spleen recognises and removes senescent red cells remain uncertain.

Within reticuloendothelial cells, the porphyrin rings of the haem portion of haemoglobin are broken down to bilirubin; the iron is released and transported to the marrow, where it is either reincorporated into newly-synthesised haem or stored in reticuloendothelial cells as ferritin or haemosiderin. The globin peptide chains are hydrolysed and their constituent amino acids re-enter the general metabolic pool.

The bilirubin is released into the blood from reticuloendothelial cells, initially unconjugated and poorly soluble, and circulates bound to albumin. In the liver, the bilirubin is conjugated and excreted in the bile.

Leucocytes and Platelets

Examination of a stained normal blood film reveals five leucocyte types: neutrophils, eosinophils, basophils, monocytes and lymphocytes, together with platelets (Fig. 1.4).

Neutrophils, eosinophils and basophils all contain conspicuous and distinctive cytoplasmic granules with specific staining characteristics which have given them their names, and whose presence has led to these leucocyte types sometimes being collectively referred to as granulocytes. Monocytes are distinguished from granulocytes by their distinctive pale blue-staining cytoplasm without conspicuous granulation (although monocytes do contain granules, these are often too small to be readily seen by light microscopy) and by their large oval or indented (sometimes horseshoe-shaped) nucleus. Most lymphocytes are smaller than the other leucocyte types, and lack specific cytoplasmic granules (they may contain a few lysosomes).

Platelets can be considered as still smaller non-nucleated cells. They are usually round or oval, and possess numerous cytoplasmic granules containing serotonin, ADP, and other factors important in haemostasis. The haemostatic function of platelets is considered further in Chapters 4 and 5.

Neutrophils

Neutrophils have more lobulated nuclei (2–5 lobes) than the other granulocytes and are therefore sometimes referred to as polymorphonuclear leucocytes (polymorphs). They are the most numerous of the

Neutrophil

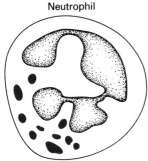

The heterogeneous cytoplasmic granules and absence of other organelles, together with the multilobed nucleus possessing heavily condensed chromatin, identify the cell. The absence of mitochondria reflects their dependence on anaerobic metabolism (cf macrophages)

Eosinophil

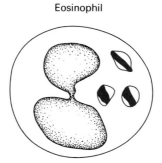

The large and distinctive cytoplasmic granules are the hallmark of the cell

Basophil

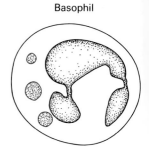

Again, distinctive cytoplasmic granules characterise the cell

Monocyte

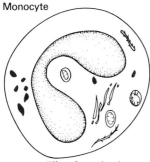

The monocyte differs from the three granulocyte types in having only small cytoplasmic granules and in possessing other cytoplasmic organelles (e.g. mitochondria, rough endoplasmic reticulum) enabling it to live in the tissues for considerable periods as macrophages

Lymphocyte

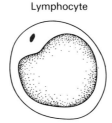

Most lymphocytes have a high nuclear-cytoplasmic ratio and lack cytoplasmic organelles apart from occasional lysosomes and mitochondria

Platelet

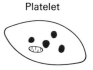

Platelets lack nuclei, their main feature is the cytoplasmic granules so important in platelet aggregation and formation of the platelet plug

Fig. 1.4 *Schematic representation of peripheral blood leuco-cytes and platelets.*

peripheral-blood leucocytes (40–75%) and their major function is the destruction of microorganisms. They function by migrating from the blood to sites of inflammation under the influence of a variety of attractant substances (chemotaxis). Once at a site of inflammation, neutrophils engulf material within a vacuole formed by invagination of the cell membrane (phagocytosis). Phagocytosed material is then killed and degraded as a result of the discharge into the phagocytic vacuole of a variety of enzymes (e.g. myeloperoxidase) and other antibacterial proteins contained within the cytoplasmic granules of the neutrophils. Phagocytosis is greatly enhanced (opsonisation) if material is coated with antibody whose interaction

with complement (see p. 12) releases complement fragments active as chemotaxins. Although microorganisms will usually be dead after phagocytosis, certain bacteria, including *Mycobacterium tuberculosis*, can survive phagocytosis (by both neutrophils and macrophages) and, in the case of macrophages (p. 8), remain viable for prolonged periods within the cell.

Neutrophils spend only a few hours in the blood before migrating into the tissues, where they probably survive a further 4–5 days, or a much shorter period if they become involved in active phagocytosis and destruction of organisms. While in the peripheral blood, neutrophils may be freely circulating (included in the blood count) or marginated along blood-vessel walls (not included in the blood count). Circulating neutrophils are derived from a physiological marrow compartment of mature granulocytes, which, when the need arises (as in infection), can be released rapidly into the circulation. This marrow reserve pool is in turn maintained by a dividing compartment of marrow granulocyte precursors (see p. 13).

Abnormalities of the peripheral-blood neutrophil count are frequently encountered in clinical medicine; qualitative defects also occur but are less frequent.

Quantitative neutrophil abnormalities

The peripheral-blood neutrophil count (see p. 21)

measures only freely circulating neutrophils. The count is therefore influenced not only by altered rates of production and destruction but also by factors affecting the distribution of cells between the different compartments outlined above. Table 1.1 sets out some of the important causes of abnormal neutrophil count in terms of the predominant mechanism involved. It should be emphasised, however, that more than one mechanism may be involved in any particular instance, and that usually the factors underlying a given mechanism are not precisely defined.

Neutrophil leucocytosis is a common clinical finding; it usually represents a non-specific response to infection, stress, or tissue damage. Most of the neutrophils

Table 1.1

Some Causes of Quantitative Neutrophil Abnormalities

Increased (neutrophilia or neutrophil leucocytosis)	Decreased (neutropenia)
Production increased	Production decreased
Chronic infections	Deficiency states
Chronic myeloid leukaemia	vitamin B_{12} deficiency
Myeloproliferative disorders	folate deficiency
Non-haematological malignancies	Drugs (especially cytotoxic agents)
	Marrow infiltrations
Distribution abnormal*	Distribution abnormal*
Acute inflammation	Acute infection†
acute infections	Viraemia
myocardial infarction	Endotoxaemia
diabetic ketoacidosis	Anaphylactic shock
Exercise and stress	
Drugs	
steroids	
adrenaline	
Destruction reduced	Destruction increased
Splenectomy	Immune causes
	SLE
	drugs
	lymphoproliferative disorders
	Hypersplenism

* Widely different mechanisms are concerned in the group of neutrophil disorders involving disordered distribution among the different neutrophil compartments. For example, acute inflammation causes neutrophilia by increasing release from the marrow reserve pool, while steroids reduce neutrophil migration from the blood.

† Acute infection leads to accelerated migration of neutrophils needed to combat infection in the tissues. The peripheral neutrophil count then depends on the response of the marrow reserve pool. Usually this response leads to normal or increased neutrophil counts, but in the early stages of infection or when the marrow reserve pool is impaired (e.g. by chronic alcoholism) neutropenia may result.

making up the leucocytosis are mature, but modest numbers of circulating precursors (i.e. a left shift in the myeloid series) may be present.

Severe neutropenia, of whatever cause, is typically associated with infection and ulceration of the mouth and perineum and with life-threatening infections by the patient's own resident flora (e.g. gram-negative gut bacteria).

Qualitative neutrophil abnormalities

Qualitative defects occur involving most aspects of neutrophil function; they arise from intrinsic defects of the neutrophil itself or from extrinsic plasma factors. Defective chemotaxis may, for example, be due to intrinsic abnormalities of the neutrophil (as in the congenital lazy-leucocyte syndrome and the myeloid leukaemias) or may be a result of plasma factors (as in diabetes mellitus). Abnormalities of phagocytosis are usually of an extrinsic nature, attributable to deficiencies of antibody and/or complement. Defective killing, on the other hand, is most often the result of an intrinsic neutrophil defect, as in chronic granulomatous disease, myeloperoxidase deficiency or Chediak–Higashi disease.

Chronic granulomatous disease is an inherited disorder which usually shows an X-linked mode of inheritance. The precise nature of the defect in this disorder is not established, but phagocytosis (organisms are readily engulfed) fails to produce the normal respiratory burst derived from the pentose phosphate pathway. As a result, little or none of the normally microbicidal hydrogen peroxidase (H_2O_2) is produced. Many microorganisms are still killed, since they generate their own H_2O_2, but if they also produce catalase (e.g. catalase-positive staphylococci) they are protected and are able to survive within the neutrophil.

Eosinophils, basophils and monocytes

Eosinophils are much less numerous than neutrophils (1–6% of leucocytes), and are readily distinguished by their large reddish-brown-staining cytoplasmic granules. The function of eosinophils is not well understood, but they are involved in IgE immune responses since they are attracted by the products of basophil and mast cell degranulation (see below) and neutralise the released inflammatory mediators. Furth-

ermore, eosinophils appear to be able to kill certain antibody-coated helminths – organisms which stimulate high levels of serum IgE.

Basophils, the least numerous (<1%) of the peripheral blood leucocytes, are identified by large violet-staining granules, which may obscure the nucleus. Tissue mast cells resemble basophils and both mast cells and basophils are able to bind specific IgE antibody (reagin) to their cell surface. Subsequent exposure to specific antigen results in rapid degranulation with release of histamine and other mediators. Type I hypersensitivity reactions (p. 19) are mediated in this way.

Monocytes (2–10%) are maturing cells that migrate into the tissues to form macrophages which function as phagocytes and as modulators of the lymphocyte-mediated immune response.

Various quantitative and qualitative abnormalities of eosinophils, basophils and monocytes/macrophages may occur. Table 1.2 sets out the important causes of

---

Table 1.2

Some Causes of Increased Circulating Eosinophils, Basophils and Monocytes

Abnormality	Important causes

Eosinophilia	Allergic disorders
	  bronchial asthma
	  allergic rhinitis
	  drug reactions
	Parasitic infection
	  e.g. gastrointestinal infestation
	Certain skin diseases
	  pemphigus, dermatitis herpetiformis
	Haematological malignancies
	  chronic granulocytic leukaemia
	  Hodgkin's disease

Basophilia	Haematological malignancies
	  chronic granulocytic leukaemia
	  polycythaemia rubra vera
	Allergic disease

Monocytosis	Haematological malignancies
	  acute and chronic monocytic
	  leukaemias
	  chronic granulocytic leukaemia
	  Hodgkin's disease
	Infections
	  subacute bacterial endocarditis
	  tuberculosis

increased numbers of these cell types in the blood. Reduction in their numbers, as well as qualitative abnormalities, have been described in a number of clinical situations, but such abnormalities are only occasionally of clinical importance. For example, in the rare lipidoses (e.g. Gaucher's disease), various lysosomal enzyme deficiencies lead to defective glycolipid degradation in macrophages. As a result, large amounts of glycolipid from senescent cells accumulate in reticuloendothelial macrophages. Since liver, spleen and bone marrow are important reticuloendothelial organs, the chronic hepatosplenomegaly and bone lesions of Gaucher's disease are easy to understand.

Lymphocytes

Lymphocytes are the most heterogeneous of the peripheral blood leucocytes; most are small with a high nucleo-cytoplasmic ratio. They are of two major types – T cells (thymus dependent) and B cells (bursa or bone-marrow dependent) – concerned respectively with cell-mediated and humoral immunity. The two cell types are not readily distinguished in peripheral-blood films, and their identification is dependent on surface-marker techniques (p. 15).

As with other haemic cell types, lymphocyte abnormalities may be either quantitative or qualitative in type.

In the interpretation of lymphocyte numbers (Table 1.3), it should be remembered that lymphocytes differ from granulocytes in several important respects. For example, many lymphocytes recirculate (i.e. re-enter the blood from the tissues) and many are long-lived (they may live for several years). In consequence, altered rates of migration can affect the blood concentration of lymphocytes without affecting the total mass of functional lymphoid tissue. In addition, short-term inhibition of lymphocyte production (e.g. by cytotoxic therapy) will not necessarily result in a reduction of the number of circulating lymphocytes. Furthermore, since circulating lymphocytes constitute only a minor proportion of the body's lymphoid tissue and are functionally heterogeneous, major lymphoid abnormalities may not be immediately apparent in the peripheral blood. For this reason, consideration of defective lymphoid function will be deferred to the section of this chapter dealing with the lymphoreticular system as a whole (p. 13). The major causes of abnormal peripheral-blood lymphocyte counts are set out in Table 1.3 (and later on in Table 1.4).

Lymphocytosis is usually due to one of the lymphoid malignancies (see Chapter 6) or to viral infection. The most important cause of virus-induced lymphocytosis is the Epstein–Barr (EB) virus, the causative agent of infectious mononucleosis.

Reduced peripheral lymphocyte counts (lymphopenia) mainly reflect reduced T-cell numbers, which may represent a primary defect (as in the immunodeficiency disorders) or may be a secondary phenomenon.

Infectious mononucleosis (glandular fever)

The disease is characterised by, and derives its name from, the presence of circulating atypical lymphocytes

---

Table 1.3

Major Causes of Abnormal Lymphocyte Counts

Increased numbers (lymphocytosis)	Reduced numbers (lymphopenia)
Certain infectious	Glucocorticoid excess
Viral (e.g. infections mononucleosis)	Therapy
Pertussis	Acute stress
Lymphoid malignancies	Malignancy
	Hodgkin's disease
	Disseminated visceral neoplasia
	Connective tissue disorders
	Certain infections
	Tuberculosis
	Cytotoxic agents
	Immune deficiency disorders

with more abundant cytoplasm than most normal lymphocytes. The cells have been shown to be T lymphocytes; these are thought to represent a secondary peripheral blood response to a primary Epstein–Barr virus infection which specifically infects, and causes proliferation of, the B cells of the lymphoid organs.

The general clinical features of the illness are those of a viraemia (e.g. headache, fever, skin rash, etc.) while its more specific features reflect the self-limited lympho-proliferation that is characteristic of the disease. Thus, cervical or generalised lymph-node and splenic enlargement (lymphadenopathy and splenomegaly) are usual findings. Virtually any organ may be involved by the viraemia, however, and liver involvement is particularly important – a mild hepatitis is common. The virus is usually transmitted by kissing and gains entry through the B-lymphoid tissues of the pharynx, hence the pharyngitis usually present.

A similar pyrexial illness with atypical lymphocytes may also be associated with cytomegalovirus or toxoplasma infection. Pharyngitis, however, is not a feature of either of these infections, and lymphadenopathy is not usually conspicuous in cytomegalovirus infection.

The detection of heterophil antibody definitively distinguishes infectious mononucleosis from other causes of atypical lymphocytosis. If any doubt remains, the demonstration of a rising titre of antibodies to EB virus will confirm the diagnosis. Heterophil antibodies are antibodies to antigens different from, and phylogenetically unrelated to, the ones which evoked the response. Thus, the heterophil antibody of infectious mononucleosis agglutinates sheep erythrocytes; this heterophil antibody forms the basis of the diagnostic Paul–Bunnell test. Other heterophil antibodies occur in normal subjects and in a variety of other clinical situations (e.g. lymphoma), but these show a different pattern of antigen reactivity. For this reason, the Paul–Bunnell test (or one of the simplified substitutes) incorporates specific antigenic absorptions designed to distinguish the heterophil antibody of infectious mononucleosis from, for example, naturally-occurring heterophil antibodies. Since the underlying lympho-proliferation of infectious mononucleosis involves antibody-producing cells (B lymphocytes), it is perhaps not surprising that unusual antibody production is not limited to heterophil antibody. Examples of other antibodies which may be produced include autoanti-

bodies causing haemolytic anaemia (p. 37) and thrombocytopenic purpura (p. 60).

There is no specific treatment for infectious mononucleosis, and the great majority of patients make a spontaneous and complete recovery. Steroids may occasionally be needed if immune phenomena such as haemolytic anaemia and thrombocytopenia cause problems, but usually only supportive therapy is indicated.

Plasma

Plasma and serum are the non-cellular fractions of anticoagulated and clotted blood respectively. Plasma contains a great many substances relevant to the whole field of internal medicine, but the ones of particular relevance to the haematologist are the coagulation factors (see Chapter 4), factors important in erythropoiesis (see Chapter 2), and the immunoglobulins (Ig – proteins having an antibody function) and complement.

Immunoglobulins

Immunoglobulins are produced by cells of the B-lymphocyte (p. 15) series, and most of the serum Ig is made by plasma cells – the terminal cells in B-cell development. When serum proteins are separated by electrophoresis, most Ig is found in the gamma-globulin fraction.

In man, there are five major structural types or classes of immunoglobulin: IgG, IgM, IgA, IgD and IgE. Antibodies formed early in the immune response (the primary response) are IgM in type, while those produced late or after repeated immunisation (the secondary response) are IgG. IgA is the main immunoglobulin in body secretions such as milk or respiratory mucus; IgD and IgE are present in the serum in only minute amounts; IgD is mainly to be found on the surface membrane of B lymphocytes, where it probably fulfils some form of recognition function; the reaginic function of IgE in the degranulation of mast cells has already been mentioned.

All immunoglobulins, regardless of class or antibody specificity, share a common basic structure which consists of two types of polypeptide chain (heavy and light chains) linked by disulphide bonds to form symmetrical four-chain molecules (Fig. 1.5). Enzymes producing limited degradation of the immunoglobulins, as well as a variety of dissociating agents affecting the disulphide and non-convalent inter-chain bonds, have been used to elucidate the structure of immunoglobulin molecules. For example, papain splits IgG antibodies into three fragments (Fig. 1.5): two fragments are identical and bind antigen (Fab – fragment antigen binding – fragments); the third fragment does not bind antigen (collectively called Fc fragments because they are obtainable in crystalline form). Amino-acid analysis of pure homogeneous proteins from different myeloma patients (p. 91) has shown that the heavy and light chains have some regions of similar amino-acid sequence (constant – C – region) and others where the amino-acid sequences show considerable variation (variable – V – region). The precise amino-acid sequence within variable regions of both heavy and light chain determines antibody specificity, while those sequences within the constant region determine distinctive biological function such as complement fixation and binding to cell-surface receptors for immunoglobulin (e.g. the receptors for the Fc of IgG on the neutrophil which enhance phagocytosis).

Serological studies of myeloma proteins have established the existence of five major types of heavy (H)

chain, each associated with one of the five major classes of Ig mentioned earlier. Light (L) chain exists in two forms (κ and λ) which can occur in combination with heavy chains of any class. However, only κ or λ light chain (not both) is found within a given Ig molecule.

IgG, IgD and IgE antibodies normally exist as monomers, each molecule having the four-chain (H_2L_2) structure outlined above. In contrast, IgM and IgA antibody usually occurs as a pentamer (($H_2L_2)_5$) or dimer (($H_2L_2)_2$) respectively, through association with a connecting polypeptide chain known as J (i.e. join) chain. Serum IgA usually exists as a monomer, while dimeric secretory IgA contains an additional secretory piece to protect it against proteolysis.

The complement cascade

Complement consists of nine serum proteins (C1–C9) which act in sequence to augment the immune defence mechanisms. The complement components are numbered in the order in which they were discovered. The complement pathway can be activated by two distinct mechanisms:

1. *the classical pathway*, in which C1 binds to the Fc region of immunoglobulin–antigen complexes and involves the sequential participation of all nine complement components;

2. *the alternative pathway*, in which the first three complement components are bypassed, with activation occurring by direct interaction of complement components with extrinsic agents such as microbial endotoxins.

The classical complement pathway

The classical pathway is outlined in Fig. 1.6. The peptide fragments C3a, C4a, and C5a are called anaphylotoxins since they stimulate the release of inflammatory mediators, such as histamine, from mast cells and basophils. Fragments C3a and C5a also act as chemotaxins (p. 12).

A number of haemic cell types, including neutrophils, eosinophils and basophils, possess receptors for C3b; interaction of antigen–antibody–C3b complexes with these receptors (immune adherence) stimulates

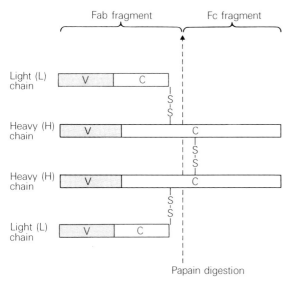

Fig. 1.5 *Schematic representation of monomeric immunoglobulin. The constant (c) and variable (v) regions of both heavy and light chains are shown, together with the approximate site of papain cleavage.*

phagocytosis of the complexes, with subsequent release of inflammatory lysozomal enzymes.

The late addition of C8 and C9 completes the cascade and gives the antigen–antibody–complement complex the property of producing cell lysis. In common with the clotting and fibrinolytic pathways, the classical complement pathway is equipped with a number of additional proteins which modulate the activation sequence. These include C1s inhibitor (p. 18) and β1H which is important in the control of C3b levels.

The alternative complement pathway

The generation of C3 convertase activity occurs without the direct participation of immunoglobulin, and is produced by the interaction of ill-defined initiating factors with two proteins, factor D (C3 proactivator convertase) and factor B (C3 proactivator protein) (Fig. 1.7). Once formed, C3b can interact with factors B and D in a positive feedback loop, and thereby form more C3b.

Whether or not the complement alternative pathway becomes an important generator activity of C3 convertase depends on competition between factor B and β1H for binding to available C3b on cell membranes. The affinity of B and β1H for C3b is greatly influenced by the presence of complex molecules in cell membranes, such as sialic acid and heparin, which increase the affinity of cell-bound C3b for β1H but not for factor B. Surfaces which are low in these structural components, such as zymogen and bacterial endotoxin lipopolysaccharides, serve as important activators of

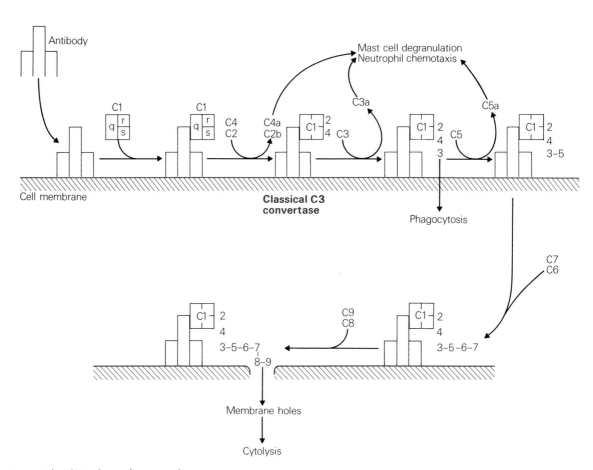

Fig. 1.6 *The classical complement pathway.*

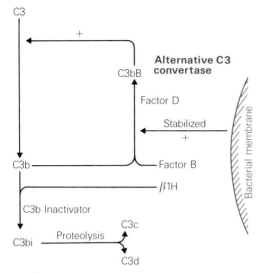

Fig. 1.7 *The alternative complement pathway.*

the alternative pathway by allowing the unregulated complexing of C3b with factor B (Fig. 1.7).

THE BLOOD-FORMING ORGANS

During adult life, blood formation (haemopoiesis) is normally confined to the axial skeleton (sternum, pelvis, sacrum, vertebrae), where approximately 50% of non-osseous material is composed of haemopoietic tissue, with fat spaces occupying the remaining marrow tissue. The bone marrow has a very large reserve capacity, and haemopoiesis can be greatly increased by expansion into the fat spaces and the non-axial skeleton. During fetal life, first the yolk sac and then the liver and spleen are major sites of haemopoiesis. Even in adults, haemopoiesis may, in certain pathological states, resume in the liver and spleen (extramedullary haemopoiesis).

Each of the peripheral blood cell types is produced by a complex sequence of maturation stages, the details of which have been the subject of much attention in recent years. Figure 1.8 and its legend set out a simplified scheme of haemopoiesis; only at a relatively late stage (Stage 4) can the different precursor forms be identified by traditional morphological methods.

Red-cell Production (Erythropoiesis)

The morphologically identifiable stages of erythroid development are characterised by progressive haemo-globinisation of cells (normoblasts) whose nuclei become increasingly degenerate and are eventually expelled to form, first, reticulocytes (p. 23) and, finally, mature red cells.

Erythropoiesis is regulated by the hormone erythropoietin and requires the presence of adequate amounts of a number of substances, including iron, vitamins B_{12} and B_6 (pyridoxine), folate, and thyroxine. Erythropoietin is produced by the interaction of a renal factor with a plasma protein, and its production (and therefore erythropoiesis) is stimulated by renal anoxia, which is in turn dependent on renal blood flow, on the Hb level, and on the precise dissociation characteristics of the oxyhaemoglobin.

White-cell and Platelet Production

Although the earliest stages of development of all leucocyte types take place in the marrow, much of the lymphocyte maturation occurs in the lymphoreticular system; immediate discussion will therefore be confined to non-lymphoid (i.e. myeloid) cell development.

The development of each of the myeloid cell types (neutrophils, eosinophils, basophils and monocytes) is characterised by progressive lobulation and chromatin condensation of the nucleus, loss of cytoplasmic RNA and other organelles, and the development of a complex complement of cytoplasmic granules.

Platelets are produced by fragmentation of the cytoplasm of very large nucleated precursors (megakaryocytes).

Leucocyte production is probably controlled by colony-stimulating factors analogous to erythropoietin.

In addition to erythroid and myeloid precursors, normal marrow also contains a number of other cell types, including plasma cells and macrophages (reticulo-endothelial cells); these cell types form part of the lymphoreticular system discussed below.

THE LYMPHORETICULAR SYSTEM

The term lymphoreticular system refers to those tissues

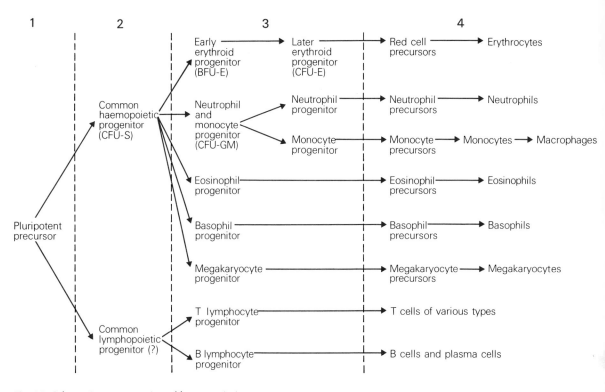

Fig. 1.8 *Schematic representation of haemopoiesis.*

Stage 1. *The existence of a pluripotent stem cell has been established in the mouse and probably also exists in man.*

Stage 2. *The existence of distinct lymphopoietic and haemopoietic progenitors in man is supported by a variety of clinical and laboratory observations. For example, proliferative disorders involving different myeloid and erythroid cell types are common, but mixed lymphoid–myeloid proliferations are very uncommon and generally follow therapy for a primary lymphoproliferative disorder. The existence of a common haemopoietic precursor was directly established by the demonstration that certain bone-marrow cells could form mixed myeloid–erythroid colonies in the spleens of irradiated mice; such cells are referred to as spleen-colony-forming units (CFU-S). The existence of a common B- and T-cell lymphoid precursor in man is controversial, and the lineages of these cells may be distinct from a very early stage.*

Stage 3. *Cells at this stage are committed to particular lineages and have become sensitive to a range of cytopoietic factors such as erythropoietin and colony-stimulating factor. In appropriate viscous culture systems, these cells are capable of forming colonies and are therefore referred to as colony-forming units. Two stages of committed erythroid progenitor have been recognised – an early progenitor forming large colonies or bursts (BFU-E) and a later cell forming smaller colonies (CFU-E). At an early stage in their development, cells of the neutrophil and monocyte series share a common progenitor (CFU-GM), but other myeloid cells seem to have distinct committed precursors from an early stage.*

Stage 4. *It is only at this stage that the different cell types can be identified by traditional morphological methods (or, in the case of lymphoid cells, by immunological methods).*

responsible for immunological competence, which depends on the complex interaction between various lymphoid-cell types and cells of the monocyte–macrophage series. The term is therefore a broad one, encompassing the familiar lymphoid organs (lymph nodes, spleen and thymus), the unencapsulated tissue lining the respiratory, alimentary and urinary tracts, and the phagocytic cells scattered throughout the body (the reticuloendothelial system).

B and T Cells and the Immune Response

Foreign material (antigen) evokes two main types of immunological response – a humoral one in which specific antibody directed against the antigen is secreted, or a cell-mediated reaction in which sensitised lymphocytes are produced. These two types of immune response are mediated by distinct sub-populations of lymphocytes – B cells (humoral immunity) and T cells (cell-mediated immunity) – which are dependent during their development on the influence of bone-marrow (or in birds, the Bursa of Fabricius) (B cells) or thymus (T cells) respectively. Once formed, both B and T cells lie dormant as non-proliferative cells of mature appearance (i.e. scanty cytoplasm and heavy nuclear chromatin) until they meet antigen. After exposure to appropriate antigen, they become large proliferating cells with an immature appearance (i.e. abundant cytoplasm and little nuclear chromatin condensation) (Fig. 1.9). After a series of cell divisions, the antigen-stimulated lymphocytes mature into the various immunological effector cells. In the case of the B-cell series, these effector cells are either memory B cells or plasma cells which, with their well-developed rough endoplasmic reticulum and Golgi apparatus, are equipped to secrete large amounts of antibody. In the case of cellular immunity, the effector T cells may either be directly cytotoxic, or influence the immune response in a positive (helper cells) or negative (suppressor cells) way, via a number of different humoral factors (e.g. helper factor, transfer factor, interferon) collectively known as lymphokines.

During much of their development, B and T cells are anatomically segregated (see below), though cooperation between these two cell types and cells of the macrophage system is essential for full immunological competence. While some simple antigens can activate B cells directly (e.g. T-lymphocyte-independent antigen), more complex antigens and the secondary immune response require the cooperation of helper T cells and macrophages (Fig. 1.9). The immune response is controlled at several levels. At the level of antigen, factors such as its rate of catabolism and sequestration affect the magnitude of the immune response. At the cellular level, the relative activities of helper and suppressor sub-populations of T cells are important. Genetic control of the immune response is mediated via a group of associated genes on the sixth chromosome, some of which determine the major histocompatibility antigens which are so important in graft rejection (p. 45).

Identification of B and T Cells

Most T cells possess localised acid phosphatase and esterase activity in suitable cytochemical preparations, but are otherwise not readily distinguishable on morphological grounds. However, T and B cell types can be differentiated by a variety of immunological surface-marker techniques. B cells are recognised by their possession of endogenous surface immunoglobulin, while T cells are identifiable by their ability to form spontaneous rosettes with unsensitised sheep erythrocytes and by their reactivity with specific anti-T-cell sera. With these techniques, approximately 70% of peripheral-blood lymphocytes can be shown to be T cells, while < 20% are B cells; the remaining cells, which have been called null cells, probably comprise a heterogeneous group of different cell types. A range of other surface structures can be identified on lymphocytes by immunological and other methods, but many such structures are shared by certain B and T cells and are therefore of less value in distinguishing between the two cell types.

Lymph Nodes

The basic structure of a lymph node is shown in Fig. 1.10. Foreign material arriving in the afferent lymph is filtered in the cortex of the node, which is composed of scattered macrophages and large numbers of B lymphocytes, frequently arranged in a follicular fashion. After antigenic stimulation, pale-staining proliferating

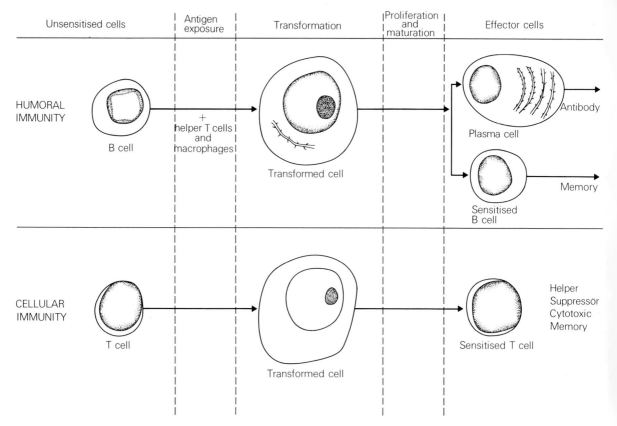

Fig. 1.9 *Simplified representation of the immune response.*

cells appear in the follicles to form germinal centres, differentiating plasma cells also appear, and mature plasma cells are seen among the lymphocytes of the medulla (a mixed B- and T-cell area). The area immediately beneath the B-cell follicles (the paracortical area) is particularly rich in T cells. Proliferation of cells in this area occurs after stimuli which provoke cell-mediated responses (e.g. grafts).

Lymphocytes enter the node either from the tissues, via the afferent lymphatics, or from the blood, via post-capillary venules. They then filter through the node to leave via the efferent lymphatics: these eventually join the thoracic duct which, in turn, drains into the venous circulation. Lymphocytes then complete their circulation by entering the tissues or recirculating through the node via the lymph node artery.

Spleen

The spleen consists of areas of lymphoid tissue surrounding blood vessels (the white pulp) and larger sinusoidal areas filled with red cells and lined with macrophages and endothelial cells (the red pulp). Within the white pulp, the area immediately surrounding the arterioles is made up principally of T cells; adjacent to this are follicular areas of B cells. Developing plasma cells are found towards the boundaries of the white pulp, extending into the red pulp.

The white pulp plays, in relation to blood-borne antigenic material, a role analogous to that served by lymph nodes in relation to lymph-borne antigen.

The red pulp of the spleen is important in the life cycle of red cells. The complex vascular channels of the red pulp offer a considerable mechanical and meta-

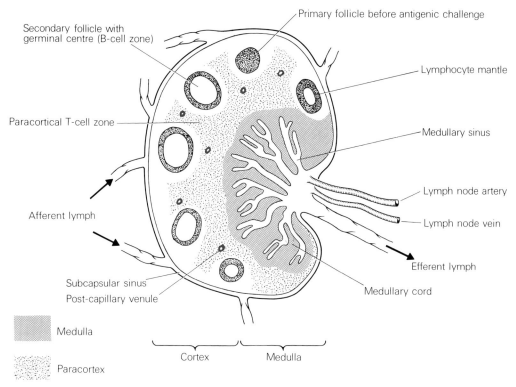

Fig. 1.10 *A normal lymph node.*

bolic obstacle to red cells traversing it, and the net result is a tendency for the red cells to lose their biconcave shape. Red cells with existing membrane or glycolytic enzyme defects are particularly susceptible to this effect and are liable to form spherocytes, which are less deformable than normal cells. As a result, their passage through the red pulp is delayed and they are liable to be phagocytosed by resident macrophages. Red cells coated with immunoglobulin are recognised by Fc receptors on the macrophages and are either completely phagocytosed or damaged, with resultant spherocyte formation. To leave the spleen, red cells must enter the splenic sinuses by passing between the lining endothelial cells. If the red cells contain a rigid inclusion (e.g. nuclear remnants or precipitated haemoglobin), this is removed (pitted) from the cell along with a portion of plasma membrane. This small portion of the cell is phagocytosed by nearby macrophages and the main part of the cell is liable to become a spherocyte.

Thymus

The thymus consists of an outer cortex densely packed with rapidly dividing lymphocytes and an inner medulla containing fewer lymphocytes. The cortical thymic cells are precursors of the functionally mature cells of the medulla, which are subsequently released into the circulation as functional T cells.

Disordered Function of the Lymphoreticular System

Under normal circumstances, the humoral and cellular arms of the immune system effectively limit the pathogenicity of invading antigen. Defects may arise at many points in the complex system outlined earlier, however, and host defence will then be compromised. In contrast, the immunological response may sometimes become excessive, resulting in a hypersensitivity state. Foreign antigen is usually responsible for hypersensitivity reactions, but occasionally self antigen is involved. Such autoimmune reactions represent a breakdown in the form of immunological tolerance (unresponsiveness) by which animals do not react immunologically to their own tissues. Well-known examples include autoimmune endocrine disease and pernicious anaemia (p. 32), autoimmune haemolytic anaemias (e.g. p. 37), and certain connective tissue disorders. The precise mechanisms involved are often poorly defined: they may arise from antigen modification (e.g. methyldopa-induced haemolysis, where the drug alters the antigenic makeup of the red-cell membrane); from antibody cross-reactivity or insertion of foreign antigen into the host-cell membrane (e.g. post-streptococcal rheumatic fever and haemolysis following mycoplasma infection respectively); or from failure of immune regulation, e.g. as a result of reduced T-suppressor cells.

In the following sections, some of the more important or clear-cut defects of humoral and cellular immunity will be described (granulocyte and monocyte/macrophage defects have already been considered), and a brief outline of the hypersensitivity states will be given.

Defective humoral immunity

Potential sites of entry of microorganisms are protected by the mechanical cleansing and bactericidal actions of secretions such as saliva, tears, mucus or urine. Interference with any of these secretions is liable to result in infection at the affected site, which then becomes a potential focus for systemic infection.

Complement, via its chemotactic properties, its binding to complement receptors on phagocytic cells, and its lytic action, plays an important role in host-defence and hypersensitivity states. Deficiency of complement components may predispose to repeated infections, and to diseases such as systemic lupus erythematosus and angioneurotic oedema (CIs inhibitor deficiency), but these deficiency states are very rare.

Antibody deficiency syndromes are less rare (Table 1.4). Specific antibody production depends on the differentiation of B cells into secreting plasma cells, which in turn often requires the help of T cells. Abnormal humoral immunity can, therefore, develop from several types of defect. Although some of these defects are rare, they have acquired a significance out of proportion to their clinical importance because of the insight they provide into the nature of the immune response.

The most common form of immune deficiency is acquired hypogammaglobulinaemia. This comprises a heterogeneous group of disorders in which the circulating B cells, though often not grossly reduced in number, have a reduced capability to form secreting plasma cells. In secondary hypogammaglobulinaemia, however, B cells and plasma cells are reduced in numbers, often by ill-defined mechanisms, in the presence of primary disorders such as malnutrition and visceral neoplasia and of immunoproliferative disorders such as multiple myeloma. Congenital hypogammaglobulinaemia is an X-linked disorder (Bruton's congenital agammaglobulinaemia) in which severe infections start to appear during the latter part of the first year of life, as IgG antibody which originated from the mother via the placenta begins to disappear.

Patients with any of these types of hypogammaglobulinaemia are subject to repeated attacks of bacterial pneumonia, gastroenteritis and septicaemia. Cell-mediated immunity, however, is normal and the patients show no increased susceptibility to viral infections. Treatment consists of vigorous use of antibiotics and regular administration of human immunoglobulin. Even with active therapy, these patients suffer frequent respiratory and gastrointestinal infections, probably because the parenterally administered human immunoglobulin does not enter the body's secretions and, in any case, contains only small amounts of IgA.

IgA deficiency, which is the commonest of the immune deficiencies affecting only a single class of Ig, is by no means rare. Antibodies to IgA are frequently demonstrable, and it is not clear whether these are a primary or secondary phenomenon. Some patients are asymptomatic, but others suffer repeated respiratory and gastrointestinal infections. Furthermore, such patients exhibit an increased frequency of malabsorption, autoimmune phenomena and allergic reactions (e.g. to IgA in blood transfusions).

Defective cell-mediated immunity

Major T-cell defects of whatever cause are characterised by a susceptibility to those infections (tuberculosis, viral and fungal infections) where host defence is primarily dependent on cell-mediated immunity. Such defects are detected clinically by reduced skin reactions to certain antigens such as tuberculin; *in vitro* they are shown by decreased numbers of cells rosetting with sheep erythrocytes, and by reduced stimulation by phytohaemagglutinin. Table 1.4 indicates some of the important causes of defective cell-mediated immunity and of combined cell-mediated and humoral deficiencies.

Table 1.4

Some Defects in Specific Host Defence Mechanisms

Defects in antibody-mediated immunity
    Late-onset (variable, acquired) hypogammaglobulinaemia
    Secondary hypogammaglobulinaemia
    Congenital hypogammaglobulinaemia
    Selective immunoglobulin deficiencies

Defects in cell-mediated immunity
    Acquired defects
        Hodgkin's disease
        Steroids
    Congenital thymic hypoplasia

Defects in both antibody and cell-mediated immunity
    Severe combined (Swiss-type) immunodeficiency
    Ataxia telangiectasia
    Wiskott–Aldrich syndrome

Hypersensitivity states

Five types of hypersensitivity reaction are recognised, each with its own characteristic immunological features.

Type I – immediate or anaphylactic hypersensitivity. This involves the interaction of specific antigens with IgE (reagin) bound to basophils and mast cells. This interaction results in the explosive degranulation of the cells, with release of a range of inflammatory mediators and chemotaxins (Fig. 1.11).

A type I allergic response may be tested for by introducing the antigen intradermally and observing the reaction over 3–5 minutes. A positive response manifests as a pruritic weal and flare reaction. Similar acute inflammatory reactions may occur in the airways in allergic asthma, in the skin in urticaria, in the nose in

allergic rhinitis and hayfever, and in the gastrointestinal tract in food allergies. In extreme circumstances an IgE-mediated reaction may spread to the circulation and produce acute cardiorespiratory failure characteristic of systemic anaphylaxis.

Type II – cytotoxic antibody-dependent hypersensitivity. Cytotoxic hypersensitivity is mediated by antibodies of the IgG and IgM classes which are directed against cellular antigens, and involves the activation of complement by the classical pathway. Cell lysis occurs by the direct membrane effects of C8 and C9 complement components (Fig. 1.6). Examples of Type II cytotoxic reactions include ABO, rhesus and autoimmune haemolytic anaemia.

A form of antibody-mediated cytotoxicity may occur when target cells are coated with only small amounts of IgG. Binding of non-sensitised lymphocytes (K cells), via the Fc portion of the IgG bound to the target cells, causes cell lysis directly. A significant proportion of the effector K cells do not have T or B cell-surface markers and fall into the category of 'null' lymphocytes. Antibody-dependent cell cytotoxicity (ADCC) operates when target cells are too large to be attacked by phagocytes.

Type III – immune complex hypersensitivity. Immune complexes are formed by the interaction of soluble antigen, circulating antibody, and complement. The release of complement fragments stimulates an inflammatory response. The eventual outcome of immune complex formation depends upon the relative concentrations of antigen and antibody. In antibody – or low antigen – excess, the complexes precipitate and are localised at the site of antigen invasion (the Arthus reaction, e.g. farmer's lung). However, when antigen is in gross excess, small soluble complexes are formed which circulate and cause widespread systemic disease (the Serum Sickness reaction, e.g. certain allergic drug reactions, systemic lupus erythematosus, etc.).

Type IV – cell-mediated or delayed hypersensitivity. Delayed hypersensitivity reactions represent an exaggerated form of cell-mediated response. The reaction is characterised by the accumulation of cytotoxic and lymphokine-producing lymphocytes with secondary recruitment of macrophages. If the antigen persists, macrophages transform to epithelioid cells and subse-

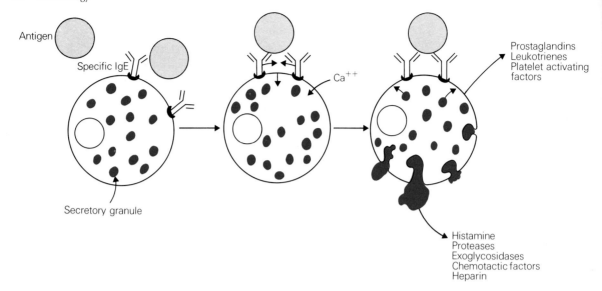

Fig. 1.11 *IgE-dependent activation of mast cells in releasing preformed and newly-generated anaphylactic mediators.*

quently to Langhans' giant cells, which form discrete granulomas. Examples of this reaction include tuberculosis and leprosy, and graft-versus-host reactions.

Type V – stimulatory hypersensitivity. In this form of hypersensitivity, the immunological response results in stimulation of the target cells. Primary thyrotoxicosis is the best example of this type.

Basic Haematological Investigation

Much haematological investigation involves the following sequence of diagnostic steps (Fig. 1.12).

The Blood Count

Automated blood count machines are now standard equipment in most hospitals. They can immediately provide a printout of the total white-blood count (WBC), platelet count and red-blood cell count (RBC), Hb, and the red-cell indices, i.e. the mean cell volume (MCV), the mean cell haemoglobin (MCH), and the mean cell haemoglobin concentration (MCHC). Coulter

electronic counters – the most widely used counters – measure the WBC, RBC, MCV and haemoglobin (Hb) level directly. The haematocrit (packed cell volume or PCV), MCH and MCHC are then derived in the following ways:

$$PCV = RBC \times MCV$$
$$MCH = Hb \div RBC$$
$$MCHC = Hb \div \text{deduced PCV}$$

Some important values are given in Table 1.5.

The different normal values for children should be noted. The Hb level of normal cord blood is higher than that of normal adult blood. Subsequently, the Hb falls to reach a nadir at about nine weeks (the normal Hb may fall as low as 9.5 g/dl). From six months to puberty, the Hb gradually rises to adult levels. Similarly, the MCV is high at birth and gradually falls to normal levels at about nine weeks.

At birth, the normal WBC is somewhat higher $(10–30 \times 10^9/l)$ than in adults, with about 60% neutrophils. During the first week of life, the neutrophil count returns to normal levels, but the WBC shows an absolute and relative lymphocytosis until the age of about four years. Platelet counts in children are similar to those in adults.

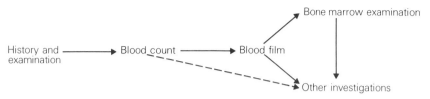

Fig. 1.12 *Haematological diagnosis.*

Table 1.5
Normal Haematological Values

ADULTS

Haemoglobin (Hb)	Men 13–18 g/dl
	Women 12–15 g/dl
Red cell count (RBC)	Men $4.5–6.5 \times 10^{12}$/l
	Women $3.8–5.8 \times 10^{12}$/l
Mean cell volume (MCV)	Adults 78–93 fl
Mean cell haemoglobin (MCH)	Adults 27–32 pg
Packed cell volume (PCV)	Men 0.40–0.52 (l/l)
	Women 0.37–0.47 (l/l)
Mean cell haemoglobin concentration (MCHC)	31–35 g/dl
Reticulocyte count	0.2–2.0%
White cell count (WBC)	Adults $5–10 \times 10^9$/l
Differential leucocyte count in absolute and in relative (brackets) numbers	Neutrophils $2.0–7.5 \times 10^9$/l (40–75%)
	Lymphocytes $1.5–4.0 \times 10^9$/l (20–45%)
	Monocytes $0.2–0.8 \times 10^9$/l (2–10%)
	Eosinophils $0.04–0.4 \times 10^9$/l (1–6%)
	Basophils less than $0.01–0.1 \times 10^9$/l (1%)
Platelet count	$150–400 \times 10^9$/l

PAEDIATRIC

Hb – cord blood	13.5–19.5 g/dl
Hb – 9 weeks	9.5–11.5 g/dl
Hb – 1 year	11–13.0 g/dl

HAEMATINIC LEVELS

Serum iron	Men 18–48 μmol/l
	Women 12–30 μmol/l
Serum TIBC	45–72 μmol/l
Serum ferritin	Men 20–250 μg/l
	Women 15–150 μg/l
Serum folate	3–15 ng/ml
Red cell folate	150–500 ng/ml
Serum B_{12}	160–1000 pg/ml

The Blood Film

Information regarding individual leucocyte types and precise erythrocyte colour, shape and size is dependent on microscopic examination of a stained blood film. The differential white-cell count (Table 1.5) is obtained by enumerating the percentages of the different leucocyte types among 100 consecutive leucocytes. The absolute count of any given leucocyte type can then be calculated from the total WBC, i.e.:

$$\text{individual leucocyte count} = \frac{\text{WBC} \times \% \text{ count}}{100} \times 10^9/\text{l}.$$

Figure 1.13 illustrates and indicates the diagnostic significance of some of the abnormalities of red-cell morphology which may be detected during examination of the blood film.

Bone Marrow Examination

This is most often performed by aspirating a small amount of tissue from the bone-marrow cavity of the sternum or posterior or anterior iliac crests. The tissue is then spread, stained and examined in the same way as peripheral blood.

Marrow examination provides information about the formation of the cellular elements of the blood. In addition, it allows an assessment of marrow, reticulo-endothelial and plasma cells, and may reveal foreign

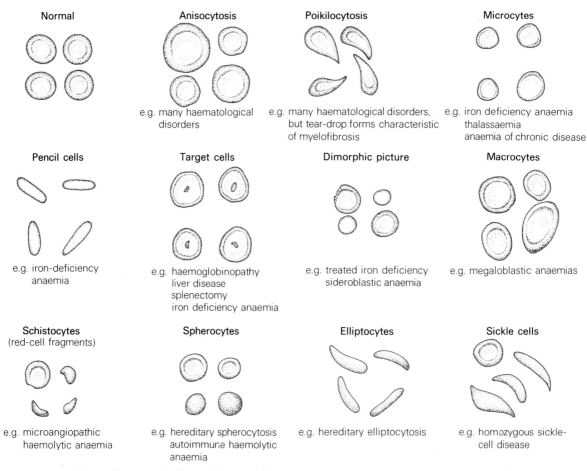

Fig. 1.13 *Some abnormalities of red-cell morphology and their diagnostic significance.*

cells such as tumour cells. An iron stain allows estimation of the patient's iron stores and incorporation of iron into the developing erythroblasts.

In general, bone marrow examination should be used to clarify the differential diagnosis suggested by clinical and peripheral blood findings. The procedure should thus be performed as a logical step in a sequence of investigations, to permit maximum information to be obtained and to make sure that potentially important additional steps such as culture for chromosomes or biopsy are not overlooked.

Where it is important to examine marrow tissue, either for foreign cells (e.g. in metastatic cancer or in Hodgkin's disease) or to establish the overall histology (e.g. in aplastic anaemia or myelofibrosis), a piece of bone may be removed from the posterior iliac crest by means of a bone-biopsy trephine needle.

Other Basic Haematological Investigations

Erythrocyte sedimentation rate

When anticoagulated blood is allowed to stand, the red cells aggregate to form cylinders of cells (rouleaux) resembling piles of plates; these then sediment, leaving a layer of clear plasma. The rate at which this process occurs is termed the erythrocyte sedimentation rate (ESR).

The ESR is primarily a measure of the tendency of the red cells to form rouleaux, which is in turn dependent on the concentration of proteins in the plasma (mainly fibrinogen, globulins and glycoproteins).

A raised ESR (normal < 20 mm/hr) provides non-specific evidence of disease. The investigation is often used to monitor disease activity during the course of an illness, and as a screening test when it is not clear whether or not a patient's symptomatology has an organic basis.

Reticulocyte count

Reticulocytes are young red cells recently released from the marrow and their numbers are raised in any condition associated with increased red-cell production. Reticulocytes are therefore raised in any haemorrhagic or haemolytic anaemia, provided the marrow is able to respond to the increased loss of red cells. If anaemia is due to decreased red-cell production, reticulocytosis will occur when the cause of the production defect is remedied (e.g. when vitamin B_{12} is given in pernicious anaemia).

A reticulocyte count is made by staining an unfixed suspension of red cells with a vital stain (one that stains living cells) such as methylene blue, preparing a blood smear from the suspension, and counting the percentage of stained red cells (reticulocytes). The term reticulocyte is derived from the fact that vital stains precipitate and stain persisting RNA in a reticular network. A quicker indication of the reticulocyte count can be obtained from a stained peripheral film by assessing the number of red cells showing a distinct basophilic tinge (i.e. polychromasia, reflecting the affinity of RNA for the basic components of the stain).

Further basic haematological investigations

Normal haematinic levels are given in Table 1.5. Subsequent chapters will indicate how further basic investigations such as Hb electrophoresis (Chapter 2), red-cell serological studies (Chapters 2 and 3) and clotting tests (Chapters 4 and 5) are used in haematological diagnosis.

2

The Anaemias

INTRODUCTION

Anaemia occurs when the haemoglobin (Hb) falls below the lower limit of the reference (normal) range for the population under study (Table 1.5, p. 21). Reference values depend mainly on age and sex. Physiological changes also occur during pregnancy, when the Hb falls because the volume of plasma increases by more than that of the red cells. Convenient values to remember for defining anaemia in well-nourished subjects living in Western countries are as follows:

adult male	< 13 g/dl
adult female	< 12 g/dl
pregnant female	< 11 g/dl

The difference in reference range for Hb between adult males and females is partly hormonal in origin and partly related to the fact that most normal women have reduced iron stores resulting from iron loss due to menstruation or pregnancy. Elderly males and females tend to have somewhat lower Hb, and no sex difference is then apparent. Values for children are given on p. 21.

Although anaemia is a common manifestation of disordered erythropoiesis, it is important to realise that erythropoiesis may be disturbed without the patient being anaemic at the time the blood sample is tested. This situation most commonly arises when the Hb is falling and anaemia is incipient, but the value is not yet actually less than the lower limit of the reference range. For example, a man whose Hb is normally 16.5 g/dl might have a fall in Hb of 3 g/dl (a definitely abnormal event, outside any possible biological variation or error in measurement), yet his Hb is still within the reference range. In some situations where erythropoiesis may be disturbed, however, the disturbance is insufficient to cause anaemia, even in the long term. The best common example of this phenomenon is seen with well-nourished alcoholics who, although not anaemic, have red-cell abnormalities suggestive of their disorder (p. 34).

Adaptations to Anaemia

Patients with anaemia may have various signs and symptoms, regardless of the specific cause for the anaemia; these will be discussed in the next sections. When describing particular types of anaemia later, any specific clinical features will then be presented.

Whether or not clinical features of anaemia become evident depends upon:

(a) The rapidity of onset and severity of the anaemia.

When anaemia develops slowly, the red cell (as a compensatory phenomenon) synthesises increased quantities of 2,3-DPG and improves oxygen delivery (p. 4, Fig. 1.2). Anaemia of rapid onset is therefore more likely to be symptomatic than if it is of slow and insidious development.

It is important to remember that 2,3-DPG is depleted when blood is stored prior to transfusion. If blood is transfused into anaemic patients, it will not be able to improve tissue oxygen delivery for a day or so.

(b) The ability of the patient to make cardiovascular compensations.

Anaemia is also compensated for by increasing cardiac output and decreasing peripheral resistance. The cardiac output is mainly increased by a larger stroke volume but there may be an element of tachycardia. Elderly patients compensate less well than younger subjects and, in consequence, become symptomatic at higher levels of Hb.

Anaemia will aggravate any pre-existing cardiovascular disease such as cardiac failure and angina pectoris.

Symptoms of Anaemia

As a general rule, young adults with chronic anaemia do not become symptomatic until the Hb falls below 8 g/dl, though elderly patients may have symptoms at 11 g/dl. Symptoms which occur are:

shortness of breath on exertion
palpitations (awareness of the heart's beat)
tiredness, weakness or fatigue.

CNS symptoms in severe anaemia, especially of the elderly, include:

faintness
giddiness
tinnitus (ringing in the ears)
headache
spots before the eyes.

Symptoms such as tiredness and weakness may be of psychological origin, particularly in young female adults; they are no commoner in chronic anaemia, when the Hb is 8–12 g/dl, than when the Hb is normal (> 12 g/dl).

Signs of Anaemia

The following signs may be seen, particularly when the anaemia is severe:

pallor of nail beds and of the mucous membranes of mouth and conjunctivae
soft ejection midsystolic murmurs
slight leg oedema (more severe if anaemia aggravates congestive cardiac failure)
retina – pallor of fundi, haemorrhages.

Treatment of Anaemia by Blood Transfusion

Wherever possible, the cause of anaemia should be identified and treatment directed at the particular cause rather than resorting to blood transfusion. There are many hazards of transfusion (see p. 49), but anaemic patients are especially apt to develop cardiac failure due to fluid overload. Vitamin B_{12} deficiency causes cardiomyopathy, and such patients may be killed by transfusion.

If the patient's anaemia cannot be treated except by transfusion, the following points should be borne in mind:

Use packed red cells, not whole blood.
Give each unit slowly, e.g. over 6 hours.
In patients with poor cardiac function give only 1–2 units/day and take i.v. drip down after each day's transfusion.
Administer short acting diuretic, e.g. frusemide.
Closely observe patient for cardiac failure (raised jugular venous pressure, crepitations at lung bases).

CLASSIFICATION OF THE ANAEMIAS

Pathophysiological Classification of Anaemia

The advantage of this approach to classification is that it provides immediate insight into the cause of the anaemia and its potential therapy. Either decreased red-cell production or increased destruction (or loss as haemorrhage) can result in anaemia. Commonly, however, these two situations coexist to some extent, since marrow disturbance often leads not only to the production of fewer cells but also to the production of defective cells which survive for a shorter period than the normal 120 days in the patient's circulation. In the classification given in Table 2.1, anaemia is categorised according to the major element producing the low Hb.

Classification of Anaemia according to Red-Cell Size

Anaemias may be classified as follows on the basis of red-cell size:

normocytic – normal sized red cells
microcytic – smaller red cells than normal
macrocytic – larger red cells than normal.

The reference range for MCV is 78 to 93 fl (p. 21), so anyone with an MCV < 78 fl has microcytosis, while an MCV > 93 fl indicates macrocytosis. Because an automated blood count, which contains a direct measurement of cell size, is a baseline investigation in most anaemic patients, this type of classification is often clinically useful. However, one of its disadvantages is that many cases of anaemia do not fall neatly into a single category.

The two types of classification, which of course are not mutually contradictory, are encompassed in Table 2.1

THE IMPORTANT ANAEMIAS

Table 2.1 lists (under *Synonyms*) the important categories of anaemia; each of these will now be considered in turn.

IRON DEFICIENCY ANAEMIA

Pathophysiology

A mixed daily diet contains 10–20 mg iron, mainly in meat, eggs, vegetables and fruit. In the presence of gastric acid, the bound iron is released and converted to the ferrous form, which is then absorbed in the duodenum and proximal small intestine. Approximately 0.5–1.0 mg of the dietary iron is normally absorbed, though more is absorbed in iron deficiency anaemia.

Iron is carried in the plasma by a specific protein, transferrin, and is stored in the tissues (bone marrow, liver, spleen) as ferritin or haemosiderin. Trace quantities of ferritin appear in plasma and are thought to give an indication of the magnitude of body iron stores.

Iron is required for production of haemoglobin, myoglobin and tissue enzymes (e.g. the cytochromes). As deficiency develops, iron is first removed from stores, then the circulating Hb is reduced, while myoglobin and cytochromes are last to be depleted (Fig. 2.1). During pregnancy, fetal iron requirements take precedence over those of the mother. Infants also require extra iron for growth.

Iron is normally lost, mainly in desquamated cells of

gut and skin, at a rate of approximately 0.5 mg/day, and normal menstrual loss averages out similarly. Thus it is easy to see how females, normally absorbing 0.5–1.0 mg/day, readily become deficient if their diet is poor, if menstruation is excessive, or if pregnancy occurs (with its additional requirement of 2 mg/day).

Aetiology

From the description of pathophysiology, most of the causes of iron deficiency will be apparent:

    poor diet
    lack of gastric acid
        achlorhydria
        gastrectomy
    malabsorption
    excessive iron requirements
        pregnancy
        infant growth
    blood loss
        excessive menstrual loss
        postmenopausal bleeding
        gastrointestinal bleeding.

Clinical Features

When taking the history and examining the patient, features may be found which reflect the aetiology of the iron deficiency (see above). There may also be brittleness of the nails (spoon-shaped nails – koilonychia – in extreme cases; Fig 2.2), angular stomatitis (Fig. 2.3) and atrophic glossitis. All these are epithelial changes which are thought to reflect deficiencies of iron-containing enzymes.

It has been claimed that iron deficiency associated with dysphagia forms a distinct syndrome, the Plummer–Vinson or Paterson–Kelly syndrome, though epidemiological surveys have not confirmed this. Dysphagia may sometimes be associated with postcricoid web formation, which is a further consequence of the mucosal atrophy caused by iron deficiency

Blood Count

As the Hb falls, the red cells become microcytic (low

Table 2.1

Characteristic Haematological Features

Disturbance	Cause	Blood	Bone Marrow	Synonyms
Decreased red-cell production	1. lack of essential nutrient			
	a. iron – depletion of stores – failure to utilise due to chronic disease	microcytic anaemia micro/normocytic anaemia	no stainable iron in marrow increased stainable iron in marrow	iron deficiency anaemia anaemia of chronic disorders
	– accumulation in mitochondria	dimorphic anaemia	ring sideroblasts, i.e. normoblasts with ring of stainable iron around nucleus	sideroblastic anaemia
	b. vitamin B_{12} c. folic acid	macrocytic anaemia macrocytic anaemia	megaloblasts megaloblasts	megaloblastic anaemia megaloblastic anaemia
	2. lack of marrow tissue a. atrophy with fatty replacement	pancytopenia	reduced cellularity	aplastic/hypoplastic anaemia
	b. replacement by fibrosis or tumour	red and white cell precursors circulating	fibrosis or tumour	leucoerythroblastic anaemia
	3. poor marrow function a. exposure to toxin, e.g. alcohol, drugs	often macrocytic	often megaloblasts	
	b. no apparent reason	variable	abnormal red-cell precursors	dyserythropoietic anaemia
Increased red-cell loss from body	acute haemorrhage	normocytic anaemia	none	
Increased red-cell destruction in body	1. normal red cell in hostile environment: a. red-cell antibodies (immune haemolysis) b. overactive splenic macrophages (hypersplenism) c. chemical exposure d. mechanical damage 2. defective red cell with poor production of: a. membrane b. enzyme (enzymopathy) c. globin – qualitative (haemoglobinopathy) – quantitative (thalassaemia)	variable	variable	haemolytic anaemia

Table 2.1 Pathophysiological classification of the anaemias. Micro-, normo- and macrocytic refer to red cells, respectively, of small, normal and large size. Dimorphic – presence of two red-cell populations, normal and microcytic. Megaloblasts – red-cell precursors with open nuclear chromatin. Pancytopenia – reduction of all circulating cellular elements.

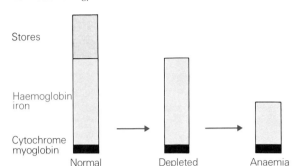

Fig. 2.1 *Distribution of iron in the body during the development of iron deficiency anaemia.*

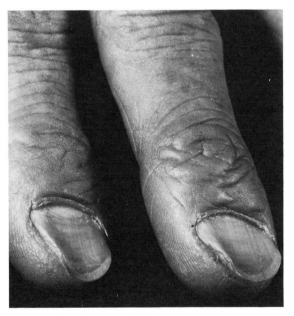

Fig. 2.2 *Koilonychia in iron deficiency.*

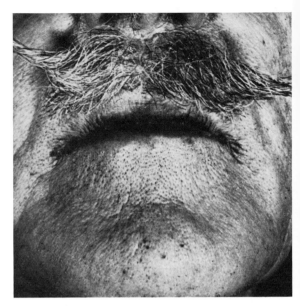

Fig. 2.3 *Angular stomatitis, a characteristic finding in iron deficiency.*

central pallor (Fig. 1.10). They also show increased variation in size (anisocytosis) and shape (poikilocytosis, Fig. 1.13), elongated or pencil cells being especially characteristic. Particularly when the iron deficiency anaemia is due to haemorrhage, there will be increased numbers of reticulocytes which are seen in the stained film as slightly larger cells of a blue-grey colour (polychromasia).

Bone Marrow

In complex cases it may be necessary to examine bone marrow. This shows erythroid hyperplasia and the normoblasts are small (micronormoblasts).

When the marrow fragments are stained for iron, stores are found to be absent, whereas in the anaemia of chronic disorders (which may also be associated with peripheral microcytosis, p. 29), the stores are usually increased.

Special Tests for Iron Deficiency

When a patient has been found to have a hypochromic microcytic anaemia, it is important to establish the cause. The differential diagnosis is usually between iron

MCV), but the red-cell count and MCHC are reduced only in the most advanced cases. The MCH and PCV are reduced in proportion to the Hb and MCV, since

$$MCH = Hb/RBC \text{ and } PCV = MCV \times RBC$$

The WBC and differential are normal. Chronic haemorrhage may increase the platelet count.

Blood Film

The red cells are microcytic and hypochromic, the hypochromia being manifest as an increased area of

deficiency, the anaemia of chronic disorders, or one of the thalassaemia syndromes (p. 39). The following investigations are of help:

a. *Serum iron, total iron-binding capacity, and transferrin saturation.* The serum iron reflects the iron being transported in plasma attached to transferrin; this is reduced in iron deficiency and also in the anaemia of chronic disorders. The total iron-binding capacity relfects the rate at which transferrin is synthesised; this tends to be increased in iron deficiency and reduced in the anaemia of chronic disorders. Therefore percentage transferrin saturation (serum iron ÷ total iron binding capacity × 100) is lower in iron deficiency than in the anaemia of chronic disease.

b. *Serum ferritin.* The level of ferritin in serum closely parallels body iron stores; it is therefore reduced in iron deficiency and normal in the anaemia of chronic diseases. The test is not available routinely in all hospitals.

c. *Studies for heterozygous thalassaemia.* In complex cases it may be necessary to exclude heterozygous thalassaemia by using appropriate investigations (p. 39). When iron deficiency coexists with heterozygous thalassaemia, the thalassaemic features may be masked, to be revealed only after iron therapy.

Establishing the Cause of Iron Deficiency

Once iron deficiency has been diagnosed, it is important to establish which of the causes (listed in the section on aetiology) are operative.

In younger females, excessive menstruation and/or repeated pregnancy are usually responsible.

In men or in post-menopausal women, iron deficiency must be considered much more seriously and it is essential to search for gastrointestinal bleeding by:

  stool examination for occult blood
  considering drug history (e.g. aspirin can cause
    bleeding)
  barium meal and follow-through
  barium enema
  endoscopy.

Therapy

Iron is best given orally as ferrous sulphate, 200 mg two or three times daily, until the Hb returns to normal and then for a further three months to replenish the iron stores. Gastrointestinal side-effects may occur, but these are not much commoner than with placebos, and are usually not troublesome. More complicated oral iron preparations offer no advantages and some disadvantages.

Iron can be given as iron dextran intravenously or intramuscularly, or as iron sorbitol citric acid complex intramuscularly. Intravenous injections may cause anaphylactic reactions, intramuscular injections may produce skin staining, and iron dextran has been shown to cause sarcomas in experimental animals. It is therefore clear that iron should only be given parenterally in the most extreme cases, e.g. patients with severe ulcerative colitis whose chronic blood loss produces a greater iron requirement than can be treated orally.

Prophylaxis

Iron deficiency during pregnancy is so common that supplementary iron should be given prophylactically. Combined preparations of iron and folic acid are of value, particularly in badly nourished populations liable to develop folic acid deficiency during pregnancy.

THE ANAEMIA OF CHRONIC DISORDERS

Patients with any chronic illness (e.g. chronic infections, connective tissue disorders, malignant disease, renal failure) tend to develop a mild anaemia which is normocytic or slightly microcytic. Usually the marrow shows increased iron stores and the serum iron and total iron-binding capacity are both low. This anaemia is unresponsive to iron therapy or to any other treatment, apart from curing the underlying disease.

SIDEROBLASTIC ANAEMIAS

The sideroblastic anaemias are a group of disorders characterised by iron accumulation in the mitochondria of the normoblast; when stained, the iron forms a ring round the nucleus, the so-called ringed sideroblast.

Some cases are hereditary and may show a response to pyridoxine. In most cases, however, the disease is acquired in later life for no known reason, or it may be secondarily associated with some other marrow disorder, antituberculous therapy or lead poisoning; these cases do not usually respond to pyridoxine and may have to be treated by transfusion.

The blood film shows two red-cell populations (dimorphic), one microcytic and hypochromic, the other of normal or even increased size. The bone marrow shows ringed sideroblasts and increased iron stores.

VITAMIN B₁₂ DEFICIENCY ANAEMIA

Pathophysiology

Vitamin B_{12} is synthesised by bacteria and is stored in significant amounts only in foods of animal origin, i.e. liver, meat, eggs, cheese and milk. A strict vegetarian diet will not supply the body's vitamin B_{12} requirement.

Proteolytic enzymes free the ingested vitamin B_{12}, which then combines with intrinsic factor secreted in the gastric juice, and the complex is absorbed in the terminal ileum. Vitamin B_{12} released into the blood from ileal cells combines with a transport protein, transcobalamin II, and is delivered to the liver stores or the bone marrow. Over 75% of the vitamin B_{12} in serum is carried by another protein, transcobalamin I, which has no known function, its bound B_{12} being unavailable to body tissues. The stores of vitamin B_{12} in the liver may last for several years even if the body has no vitamin B_{12} intake.

There is still considerable speculation about how vitamin B_{12} deficiency causes anaemia, but it is likely that its depletion interferes with the normoblast's nucleic acid metabolism.

Aetiology

From a knowledge of pathophysiology, most of the causes of vitamin B_{12} deficiency can be listed as follows:

strict vegetarian diet
lack of gastric intrinsic factor
   gastric atrophy in pernicious anaemia
   total gastrectomy
   some cases of sub-total gastrectomy
malabsorption
   stagnant loop syndromes
   ileal resection and Crohn's disease
   fish tapeworm
   other causes.

Clinical Features

Manifestations reflecting the aetiology of vitamin B_{12} deficiency may be apparent and there is often an atrophic glossitis (Fig. 2.4). Deficiency of vitamin B_{12} also has neurological effects, the most important of these being peripheral neuropathy and subacute combined (posterior and lateral column) degeneration of the spinal cord. The patient may complain of paraesthesiae, and sensory loss may be apparent on testing.

Blood Count

The anaemia of vitamin B_{12} deficiency is macrocytic, and in early cases the MCV may be raised (macrocytosis) while the haemoglobin is still normal. The MCHC is unchanged, and the platelet count is usually reduced, together with the WBC and the percentage of neutrophils. Since vitamin B_{12} deficiency depresses the red and white cells as well as the platelets, it may be said to cause a pancytopenia.

Blood Film

The red cells are macrocytic and there is anisocytosis, (variation in cell size) and poikilocytosis (variation in cell shape) (Fig. 1.13). An increased number of lobes is seen in the nucleus of the neutrophil, a phenomenon known as hypersegmentation (also sometimes referred to as a right shift in the neutrophil series). Fewer platelets than normal may be observed.

Bone Marrow

It is usual to examine the bone marrow when vitamin B_{12} deficiency is suspected. The marrow shows an increase in red-cell precursors (erythroid hyperplasia), many of which are large and possess abnormal nuclei (megaloblasts). Granulocytopoiesis is also disordered and giant immature neutrophils (giant metamyelocytes) may be seen.

Special Tests for Vitamin B_{12} Deficiency

Macrocytic anaemia with a megaloblastic marrow may also be caused by folic acid deficiency and a number of other disorders. The following investigations are useful for differentiation:

a. *Serum B_{12}*. In spite of the fact that most of the vitamin B_{12} in serum is bound to transcobalamin I and has no known function, a low level of serum B_{12} is a fairly good indicator of deficiency, although low values can also be found in folic acid deficiency. In a small proportion of patients with vitamin B_{12} deficiency, the serum B_{12} may be normal.

b. *Serum and red-cell folic acid*. The level of folic acid in serum closely reflects recent dietary intake and many hospital patients have low levels. Folic acid in the red cells reflects folate status over a much longer period and, while low levels are to be expected in folate deficiency, they can also occur in vitamin B_{12} deficiency.

c. *Deoxyuridine suppression test*. This is a test to assess nucleic acid metabolism in bone marrow. Abnormal results are found in megaloblastic anaemia and, by attempting to correct the abnormality with vitamin B_{12} or folic acid *in vitro*, it is possible to discriminate between the two deficiencies. Unfortunately, the test is too complex for routine use.

From the above discussion it will be apparent that it is sometimes difficult to establish whether a patient is vitamin B_{12} or folic acid deficient. The differentiation is fairly simple if the serum B_{12} is low and the red cell folate

normal or, of course, vice versa. Sometimes, however, the diagnosis of vitamin B_{12} deficiency cannot be established until the cause of the deficiency has been determined.

Establishing the Cause of Vitamin B_{12} Deficiency

The clinical features may indicate the cause of the deficiency (poor diet, gastric or ileal resection) but further investigation will still be required:

a. *Intrinsic-factor and parietal antibodies*. The gastric atrophy of pernicious anaemia is thought to be autoimmune, and circulating antibodies to intrinsic factor and parietal cells are indeed found in the vast majority of pernicious anaemia patients. Intrinsic factor antibodies are rarely found in the absence of pernicious anaemia but parietal cell antibodies are common in the elderly.

b. *Schilling test*. This is a test of vitamin B_{12} absorption in which radioactive cyanocobalamin (^{57}Co or ^{58}Co) is given orally at the same time as a large 'flushing' non-radioactive dose is given intramuscularly. The flushing dose is intended to block the circulating transcobalamins; any absorbed radioactive vitamin B_{12} will therefore circulate unbound and be excreted in the urine, which is then collected and counted. The flushing injection also prevents uptake of radioactive vitamin B_{12} by the liver. This is important because the long period of liver storage would lead to a high radiation exposure.

Since the flushing injection partially treats any vitamin B_{12} deficiency, before this procedure is carried out it is important to ensure that the marrow aspiration has already been performed and that a sample has been obtained for vitamin B_{12} assay.

The Schilling test is normally performed in two separate parts. In Part I, radioactive vitamin B_{12} alone is given orally, while in Part II it is given with intrinsic factor. As one might expect, the results in Parts I and II are normal in nutritional deficiency and low in intestinal malabsorption. In intrinsic factor deficiency, the Part I result is low and the Part II is normal.

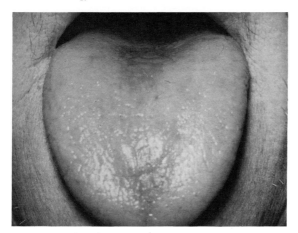

Fig. 2.4 *Atrophic glossitis in pernicious anaemia.*

Pernicious Anaemia

This is the commonest cause of vitamin B_{12} deficiency and occurs predominantly in the elderly. An auto-immune gastritis, evidenced by antibodies to intrinsic factor and parietal cells, leads to loss of gastric intrinsic factor and to typical results in the Schilling test. The gastric atrophy predisposes to gastric carcinoma and patients may require appropriate gastrointestinal investigation. Since the parietal cell produces acid as well as intrinsic factor, the atrophy leads to achlorhydria,

although there is little point in performing gastric function tests to confirm this.

Pernicious anaemia may also be complicated by other autoimmune diseases such as myxoedema.

Therapy and Therapeutic Response

Intramuscular injections of hydroxocobalamin (250 μg) are given monthly. It is possible to give injections somewhat less frequently but they then tend to be forgotten altogether.

The response of deficient patients to vitamin B_{12} is much faster than the treatment of iron deficiency and the patient may feel better after only 24–48 hours. The level of reticulocytes rises in the blood (Fig. 2.5) and should be monitored as an early sign of response.

Folic acid, in pharmacological doses, will correct the haematological effects of vitamin B_{12} deficiency, but the neurological complications will continue to develop. For this reason it is absolutely essential to ensure that no patient who really has vitamin B_{12} deficiency is mis-diagnosed and treated with folic acid.

Vitamin B_{12}-deficient or folic acid-deficient patients will respond specifically if the appropriate vitamin is given as a therapeutic trial in very low daily doses. This approach is not suitable for routine use.

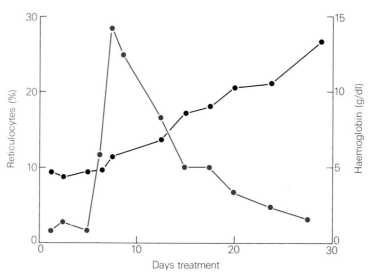

Fig. 2.5 *Reticulocyte response and rise in haemoglobin following vitamin B_{12} treatment in pernicious anaemia.*

FOLIC ACID DEFICIENCY ANAEMIA

Pathophysiology

Folic acid is present in vegetable as well as animal foods, but it is readily destroyed by cooking. Absorption is in the more proximal small intestine, and storage in the liver is sufficient to last only a few months if intake ceases.

Folic acid functions as a coenzyme in a number of important reactions. Its involvement in nucleotide synthesis is particularly important. Deficiency therefore interferes with nucleic acid synthesis, but the exact mechanism by which folic acid deficiency causes anaemia is not known.

Aetiology

Causes of folic acid deficiency are listed below:

    poor diet
    malabsorption
        gluten sensitivity
        tropical sprue
        post-gastrectomy
        other causes
    increased requirements
        pregnancy
        haemolytic anaemia
    folic acid antagonists
        methotrexate (antimitotic drug)
        pyrimethamine (antimalarial)
        co-trimoxazole
        possibly anticonvulsants.

The aetiological factors listed above are straightforward, with the exception of anticonvulsant drugs. It has not been proved that folic acid deficiency is the cause of the macrocytosis found in patients taking anticonvulsants, but there is no doubt that such patients do become macrocytic and develop low red-cell folate levels.

Clinical Features

There may be an atrophic glossitis but, in contrast to vitamin B_{12} deficiency, no well-defined neurological lesions are recognised in folic acid deficiency.

Routine Tests

Blood count, blood film, and bone marrow show the same features as in vitamin B_{12} deficiency.

Special Tests for Folic Acid Deficiency

See special tests for vitamin B_{12} deficiency (p. 31).

Establishing the Cause of Folic Acid Deficiency

If clinical features do not point to the aetiological factor, it is usually necessary to investigate the patient for malabsorption syndrome. Cases of gluten sensitivity often present as macrocytic anaemia due to folic acid deficiency.

Therapy and Therapeutic Response

Whether or not the patient is malabsorbing, it is usually possible to treat with oral folic acid, 5 mg daily. Parenteral therapy with folinic acid must be given to reverse the effect of folic acid antagonists.

The therapeutic response should be rapid, with a reticulocytosis.

Prophylaxis

It is sensible to give prophylactic folic acid to pregnant women, particularly if their diet is poor.

APLASTIC OR HYPOPLASTIC ANAEMIA

This type of anaemia results from aplasia or hypoplasia of the marrow. The anaemia is often associated with a low WBC and platelet count (pancytopenia).

Aetiology

Some cases of aplastic anaemia may arise for no known reason, while other cases are known to be secondary to:

overdosage of antimitotic drugs
idiosyncratic reaction to drugs, e.g. chloramphenicol, gold, and other anti-inflammatory agents
viral hepatitis
radiation.

Some types (e.g. Fanconi's anaemia) are usually diagnosed during childhood.

Clinical Features

There are no specific features associated with anaemia due to aplasia. If, however, there is depression of the neutrophils there will be a tendency to infection, and depression of the platelets will lead to haemorrhage; these clinical features are similar to those found in acute leukaemia (p. 82).

Blood Count

The anaemia is normocytic or slightly macrocytic. The WBC and platelet count may also be low.

Blood Film

The red cells show anisocytosis and poikilocytosis and may be slightly macrocytic. There may also be an associated reduction in white cells and platelets.

Bone Marrow

When marrow is aspirated, the most important feature is a reduction of cellularity. Cellularity may vary widely from area to area, however, and trephine biopsy is needed for a better assessment.

Therapy

It is important to remove any factors which may have caused the aplasia and to give supportive treatment for anaemia (packed red-cell transfusion), neutropenia (antibiotics and possibly leucocyte transfusion), and thrombocytopenia (platelet transfusion).

Curative treatment is only rarely possible, e.g. by bone marrow transplantation from an identical twin or HLA-compatible sibling donor. Androgens and corticosteroids have been employed, but their benefits have never been proven by clinical trial.

Prophylaxis

Care must be taken to monitor and minimise radiation exposure. Drugs such as chloramphenicol which regularly cause aplasia should never be prescribed if there is a practicable alternative. Anti-rheumatic and other drugs that occasionally cause aplasia should be prescribed only if the patient's blood count is carefully monitored.

LEUCOERYTHROBLASTIC ANAEMIA

This anaemia is characterised by the presence of white-cell and red-cell precursors in the peripheral blood. Myelofibrosis (p. 88) or infiltration of marrow by myeloma or carcinoma may be responsible.

EFFECTS OF ALCOHOL ON THE BLOOD

Alcohol is a marrow toxin which often causes macrocytosis without anaemia. Acute exposure to large quantities of alcohol can cause thrombocytopenia.

Nutritional folic acid deficiency may be a complicating factor in alcoholics, although it is relatively unusual in Britain.

DYSERYTHROPOIETIC ANAEMIA

The term dyserythropoiesis refers to abnormal erythroid maturation in the marrow, which is of normal or increased cellularity but fails to produce sufficient red cells. Morphological manifestations include abnormalities of cell size and shape and abnormalities of nuclear appearance.

Some dyserythropoiesis is evident in most anaemias, but it may be a dominant feature in some of the preleukaemic syndromes and in erythroleukaemia.

The congenital dyserythropoietic anaemias are a poorly-understood group of hereditary refractory anaemias, generally discovered early in life, in which dyserythropoietic changes are the dominant feature of the bone marrow.

HAEMOLYTIC ANAEMIA

Pathophysiology

The flexibility of the red cell is the major feature determining how long it remains in the circulation. At the end of its normal 120-day lifespan the red cell, having become too rigid to pass through the sinusoids of the spleen, liver and marrow, is phagocytosed by the reticuloendothelial system. In most haemolytic anaemias the red cells become inflexible prematurely and are then removed from the circulation by the reticuloendothelial system: this is termed extravascular haemolysis. Occasionally the red cells are actually lysed in the circulation: this is intravascular haemolysis.

During intravascular haemolysis, haemoglobin is released into the circulation. This also occurs, though to a lesser extent, with extravascular haemolysis. Haemoglobin released into the circulation combines with haptoglobin and is then rapidly removed from the circulation, mainly by the liver. Since the haptoglobin does not recirculate, its level in the plasma is reduced by haemolysis. If intravascular haemolysis is excessive, more haemoglobin is released than can combine with haptoglobin, and free haemoglobin circulates in the plasma. Some is excreted in the urine, visible as haemoglobinuria, while some of its iron is deposited in renal tubular cells as haemosiderin. Renal haemosiderosis does not cause functional impairment but, in time, desquamation of renal tubular cells occurs and may be detected as haemosiderinuria. Excessive intravascular haemolysis can cause acute renal failure because of tubular necrosis.

The haemoglobin released from damaged cells is broken down to bilirubin, which passes to the liver for conjugation. An unconjugated hyperbilirubinaemia occurs if the liver is unable to conjugate the bilirubin produced. The excess bilirubin production is reflected by raised faecal urobilinogen. Urinary urobilinogen, which is more readily detected, is also raised.

In chronic haemolysis, the excessive production of bile pigments may lead to pigment stone formation within the biliary system. This can then cause an obstructive jaundice in addition to the haemolytic jaundice.

As a compensatory response to haemolysis, the bone marrow undergoes erythroid hyperplasia and an increased percentage of reticulocytes is found in the peripheral blood.

Clinical Features

The main clinical feature pointing to haemolytic anaemia is a mild jaundice. In certain chronic congenital anaemias, the erythroid hyperplasia in the marrow affects the shape of the facial bones and a typical facies may be seen. Haemoglobinuria may be noted with intravascular haemolysis. There may be clinical features associated with particular types of haemolytic anaemia, which will be described later.

Blood Count

There may be changes associated with specific haemolytic anaemias (see below) but in general the anaemia is normocytic or slightly macrocytic.

Blood Film

There will probably be features indicative of the cause of the haemolytic anaemia (see below), as well as polychromasia if the reticulocyte count is raised.

Bone Marrow

This will usually show erythroid hyperplasia.

Special Tests

From the description of the pathophysiology, the following changes might be expected.

Reticulocytosis

This feature is a secondary consequence of haemolysis. If the bone marrow fails to respond, an aplastic crisis may develop in which the Hb falls rapidly without a corresponding reticulocytosis. Infections may precipitate such marrow failure, which is usually temporary.

Hyperbilirubinaemia

Haemolytic anaemia is typically associated with an unconjugated hyperbilirubinaemia, but this may not be evident if the haemolysis is mild and the liver is functioning well. Newborn babies, on the other hand, particularly those who are premature, have poor hepatic conjugating ability. If they have a haemolytic anaemia, there is no jaundice *in utero* because the bilirubin crosses the placenta, but after birth the bilirubin (including the unconjugated form) rises rapidly and may cause kernicterus (p. 51).

Reduced haptoglobin

This is particularly evident with intravascular haemolysis, though it is also found with extravascular haemolysis.

Red-cell survival

All the features of haemolysis listed above are secondary phenomena, and it may occasionally be difficult to establish that haemolysis is occurring. In these circumstances it is necessary to study the patient's red-cell survival to assess whether or not it is shortened. This technique involves removing blood from the patient, labelling the red cells with radioactive chromium (⁵¹Cr) and reinjecting them into the patient's circulation. Blood samples are taken at intervals thereafter and the results plotted (Fig. 2.6). It should be noted that in normal subjects the radioactivity decreases more rapidly than one might expect for a red-cell survival of 120 days; this is due to slight elution of radioactivity

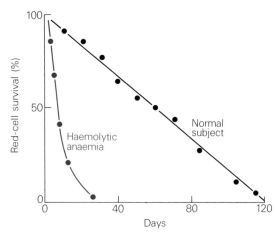

Fig. 2.6 *Red-cell survival curve showing shortening due to haemolytic anaemia.*

from the circulating red cells. Nevertheless, by establishing a normal range it is easy to assess whether the results in the patient reflect a shortened or normal red-cell survival.

Surface counting

When the red-cell survival test is in progress, the ⁵¹Cr released from destroyed cells tends to accumulate in the liver or the spleen or in both. This radioactivity, if excessive, can be detected by locating an isotope counter over these organs. Such measurements may sometimes be useful in assessing further treatment. If, for example, no radioactivity accumulates in the spleen, there may be little benefit from removing this organ in an attempt to minimise the haemolysis.

Stool radioactivity

While chronic blood loss by haemorrhage will eventually produce iron deficiency anaemia, initially a normocytic anaemia with a raised percentage of reticulocytes may be seen. Such cases may be confused with cases of haemolysis, particularly if occult blood testing has been negative. Red-cell survival will also be shortened but the correct diagnosis can be established by demonstrating the presence of ⁵¹Cr in the stools.

Establishing the Cause of the Haemolytic Anaemia

The various causes of haemolytic anaemia are listed in Table 2.1. These will now be considered individually and specific features discussed.

Red-cell antibodies

Most red-cell antibodies that cause haemolysis are autoimmune, i.e. produced by the patient against his own red cells. Antibodies are either of the IgG or IgM type.

IgG antibodies usually react best at 37°C (warm antibodies), and they coat the red cell. The macrophages first remove some red-cell membrane containing the bound antibody, but without significantly decreasing the volume of the cell so that it is therefore forced to become spherocytic (Fig. 1.10). Once the cell is spherocytic, it becomes too rigid to pass through the sinusoids and is phagocytosed (extravascular haemolysis). This is what happens in most autoimmune haemolytic anaemias, whether they are of the idiopathic type, or secondary to drug therapy (especially α-methyldopa) or to systemic lupus erythematosus or another disease.

Rarely, IgG antibodies react better at temperatures below 37°C (cold antibodies) and this can happen *in vivo* when the extremities are cold. When these coated cells reach a warmer part of the body, the antibody may, by the complement mechanism, lyse the red cell intravascularly. This disorder is termed paroxysmal cold haemoglobinuria.

IgM antibodies react best in the cold. They usually cause agglutination of the red cells, and this phenomenon is often suspected from the fact that *in vitro* it causes an artificial elevation of the MCV. *In vivo*, red-cell agglutinates may form in cold extremities, causing Raynaud's phenomenon and even gangrene. This disorder is termed cold haemagglutinin disease.

The possibility of autoimmune haemolytic anaemia may be suspected when spherocytes are seen in the film, and the diagnosis is confirmed by the Coombs or antiglobulin test (p. 42).

The basic operation in the Coombs test is to add an animal antibody against human γ-globulin to the red cells suspected of carrying bound autoantibody. When the red cells have been removed from a patient with an autoimmune haemolytic anaemia, they will react *directly* by agglutination. If the level of antibody is high, it may also be detectable in serum by performing the Coombs test *indirectly*. In this case, the patient's serum is first mixed with suitable donor red cells; the donor cells bind any autoantibody and can then be agglutinated by addition of the antibody to human γ-globulin.

Autoimmune haemolytic anaemia is treated by removing any possible cause. Many cases remit spontaneously or are too mild to merit therapy. In severe cases, corticosteroids may be of benefit, and it is sometimes necessary to resort to splenectomy.

Haemolytic disease of the newborn

This is an alloimmune haemolytic anaemia caused by transfer of maternal antibody across the placenta (p. 51).

Hypersplenism

The term hypersplenism refers to the fact that substantial splenomegaly of any cause may be associated with anaemia, neutropenia, or thrombocytopenia in any combination. A number of mechanisms may contribute to the cytopenias. These include increased activity of splenic macrophages, simple anatomic sequestration, and increased plasma volume. When marrow function is not compromised, splenectomy will be of benefit.

Chemical exposure

Drugs (e.g. phenacetin and sulphonamides) and chemicals (e.g. lead) can damage the red cells directly and cause a haemolytic anaemia.

Mechanical damage

This can be due to artificial materials (e.g. prosthetic heart valves), to fibrin strands in the vessels (microangiopathic haemolytic anaemia), or to repeated compression of blood vessels in the feet by marching or running (march haemoglobinuria).

Red-cell membrane abnormalities

Important specific disorders in this group of haemolytic anaemias include hereditary spherocytosis, hereditary elliptocytosis and paroxysmal nocturnal haemoglobinuria.

Hereditary spherocytosis and elliptocytosis are usually inherited as autosomal dominant characteristics and are readily recognised by their characteristically-shaped red cells in the blood film (Fig. 1.10). The spherocytosis of hereditary spherocytosis is differentiated from that of an autoimmune haemolytic anaemia by a family history and a negative direct Coombs test. An osmotic fragility study may also be of help by showing the typical findings of hereditary spherocytosis (Fig. 2.7). Treatment is by splenectomy, which prolongs

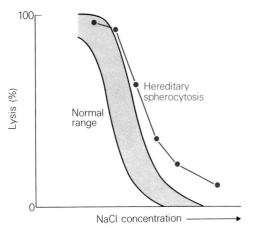

Fig. 2.7 *Osmotic fragility curve. When red cells are suspended in low concentrations of sodium chloride (NaCl) they swell, first becoming spherical and then lysing. The relationship between percentage lysis and NaCl concentration is sigmoid. In hereditary spherocytosis, many of the cells are already spherical and lyse rapidly at low NaCl concentrations, so the percentage lysis is greater than normal at a given NaCl concentration.*

red-cell survival and reduces the frequency of complications (e.g. aplastic crises, gallstones).

Paroxysmal nocturnal haemoglobinuria is a rare, acquired, chronic intravascular haemolytic anaemia, in which the red cells do not display any characteristic abnormality of shape but are abnormally sensitive to lysis by complement. Detection of this defect forms the basis of diagnostic tests such as Ham's acid lysis test and the sucrose haemolysis test. Chronic loss of iron

through haemosiderinuria frequently leads to iron deficiency. In addition to anaemia, patients may have neutropenia, thrombocytopenia and recurrent thromboses, and reactions to blood transfusions may be troublesome.

Enzymopathy

Glucose 6-phosphate dehydrogenase (G6PD) deficiency is the commonest abnormality of the red-cell enzymes. The enzyme deficiency is transmitted by a mutant gene on the X chromosome. Affected males manifest full expression of the defect, as do homozygous women. In heterozygous women, because one of the two X chromosomes is randomly inactivated (the Lyon hypothesis), half the red cells have a normal complement of G6PD, while half are defective. It is clear, therefore, that the severity of the defect in G6PD deficiency may vary greatly and that *in vitro* demonstration of reduced enzyme activity reflects varied and complex genetic abnormalities.

G6PD deficiency results in reduced aerobic pentose phosphate pathway activity, with consequent reduction of NADPH production and reduced protection against oxidation of sulphydryl groups (p. 4). This may result in denaturation and precipitation of Hb, and damage to the red-cell membrane, with subsequent reduction in red-cell life span. Usually, this reduction is only slight and the marrow readily compensates to produce normal peripheral erythroid values. However, patients with G6PD deficiency are unable to withstand any abnormal oxidative stress (e.g. certain drugs such as primaquine and phenacetin, or the ingestion of fava beans—favism), and acute haemolysis ensues.

Pyruvate kinase (PK) deficiency, which shows an autosomal recessive inheritance, leads to failure of ATP formation and accumulation of 2,3-DPG (p. 4). The former causes haemolysis, while the increase of 2,3-DPG lowers oxygen affinity and decreases the marrow response. Patients with PK deficiency therefore have haemolysis with gross anaemia, but the oxygen supply to the tissues is maintained by the low oxygen affinity.

Haemoglobinopathy

The term is used to describe conditions in which an abnormal haemoglobin is produced, the most common being sickle haemoglobin (HbS) in Negroes, Indians and Arabs (Table 2.2). The HbS molecule has an abnormal β chain, β_s, in which one amino acid differs from normal. When exposed to low oxygen tensions, the molecule comes out of solution and forms large crystals which deform the red cell into a rigid sickle (Fig. 1.10). This leads in turn to haemolysis and may block blood

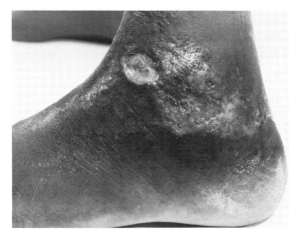

Fig. 2.8 *Leg ulcers in sickle-cell disease.*

Table 2.2

Features of the Common Haemoglobinopathies and Thalassaemias

	Heterozygote	*Homozygote*
Sickle-cell anaemia		
Blood film	normal	sickle cells
Special tests	sickle test positive	sickle test positive
β-thalassaemia		
Blood film	microcytes and target cells (Fig. 1.13)	microcytes and normoblasts
Special tests	raised HbA$_2$ ($\alpha_2\delta_2$)	Hb mainly HbF ($\alpha_2\gamma_2$)
α-thalassaemia		
Blood film	normal or microcytic	normoblasts (hydrops fetalis)
Special tests	globin chain synthesis studies	globin chain synthesis studies

---

vessels, resulting in painful infarcts in any part of the body (sickle crises). Leg ulcers may arise in infarcted areas of skin (Fig. 2.8).

Homozygous disease (sickle-cell anaemia) presents the clinical picture of severe haemolytic anaemia punctuated by crises, which may occur at any time but especially when the patient is infected.

Heterozygotes (sickle-cell traits) usually display no haematological abnormalities and are well unless rendered severely anoxic, e.g. by anaesthesia. For this reason, before giving a general anaesthetic it is mandatory to establish whether any Negro, Indian or Arab is a heterozygote by requesting a sickle screening test.

Thalassaemias

This group of disorders is characterised by failure to synthesise normal quantities of haemoglobin. Adult haemoglobin, $\alpha_2\beta_2$, is most commonly affected, and the disorder is termed α- or β-thalassaemia, depending upon which chain is synthesised in reduced quantities. The α-type is common in the Far East and the β-type in the Mediterranean countries. The homozygous forms are the most serious (Table 2.2); the β-type causes a transfusion-dependent anaemia (and, eventually, manifestations of iron overload; p. 49) and the α-type causes either hydrops fetalis or chronic haemolytic anaemia (haemoglobin-H disease), depending on the exact pattern of inheritance.

The heterozygous forms cause only a very mild anaemia. This requires no therapy except during pregnancy or serious illness, when the marrow is unable to increase its activity as much as can the marrow of a normal person, and transfusion may be required. It is important to distinguish the heterozygous thalassaemias from iron deficiency since they both cause microcytosis.

Antenatal diagnosis of homozygous thalassaemia is possible; the mother may then be offered a termination of pregnancy.

3

Blood Transfusion

INTRODUCTION

Transfusion practice today is orientated towards giving the patient the component of blood best suited to his particular needs. This leads to better replacement therapy and more economical use of blood, which is a limited resource. On occasion, it may be necessary to remove abnormal cells (exchange transfusion) or plasma components (therapeutic plasmapheresis) and replace them with normal blood components.

The other principal aspect of blood transfusion is concerned with the immunological consequences. The cells and proteins of the blood carry antigenic determinants which are polymorphic, i.e. present in some individuals and not in others. Thus, a blood transfusion may immunise the recipient against donor antigens which he lacks (i.e. alloimmunisation), and repeated transfusions will increase the chance of this happening. Similarly, the transplacental passage of fetal cells during pregnancy may alloimmunise the mother against incompatible fetal antigens inherited from the father. The alloantibodies so formed are responsible for most of the immunological problems encountered in blood transfusion therapy, and for alloimmune neonatal cytopenias.

RED-CELL ANTIGENS AND ANTIBODIES

The discovery of the ABO system by Landsteiner in 1900 marked the beginning of safe blood transfusion. Since then a number of other blood group systems have been discovered; these include the Rhesus (Rh),

Kell, Duffy, Lewis and Kidd systems. The clinical importance of a blood group antigen depends on the frequency of occurrence of the corresponding antibody and its ability to haemolyse red cells *in vivo*. On these criteria, the ABO system is easily the most important, followed by the Rh system.

ABO System

This system is defined by three genes, A, B and O, on chromosome nine, which are inherited in pairs as Mendelian dominants (Table 3.1). The A and B genes code for specific enzymes which convert a precursor substance (the H antigen) into A and B antigens respectively. The O gene is amorphic, i.e. it has no effect and the H antigen persists unchanged in group O

Table 3.1

ABO Blood Group System

Blood group (phenotype)	Genotype	Red cell antigens	Antibodies	Frequency in UK (%)
O	OO	(H)*	anti-A + anti-B	46.7
A	AA/AO	A	anti-B	41.7
B	BB/BO	B	anti-A	8.6
AB	AB	A + B	none	3.0

* Although the H antigen is the precursor substance for enzymes encoded by A and B genes, it is genetically independent.

persons. It is unnecessary to elaborate on finer points of the ABO system (e.g. A_1 and A_2 subgroups), which are of minor clinical significance.

Antigens A, B and H have variable expression on most cells, including leucocytes and platelets. These antigens are also present, in water-soluble form, in most body fluids in about 80% of the population who have inherited the secretor gene.

A feature of the ABO system is the natural occurrence of anti-A and anti-B, in the absence of the corresponding red-cell antigens (Table 3.1), without any obvious immunising stimulus such as blood transfusion or pregnancy. These antibodies are detectable after the age of about three months and it is thought that exposure to environmental A and B antigenic material (possibly of bacterial or viral origin via the gastrointestinal tract) provides the immunising stimulus.

The Ig class of anti-A and anti-B, whether 'naturally occurring' or immune, seems to depend on the ABO group of the individual. In group A and B subjects, anti-B and anti-A are wholly or predominantly IgM, but in group O subjects they are often partly IgG, especially after immunisation. Immune anti-A and anti-B, whether IgM or IgG, lyse A and B cells more readily than the naturally-occurring antibodies. In this respect, the naturally-occurring antibodies react best at 4°C, whereas the immune antibodies react at 37°C, and may therefore activate complement more efficiently. Group O donors should always be screened for anti-A and anti-B immune haemolysins, which may cause haemolysis when group O whole blood is transfused to recipients with A and/or B antigens. These dangerous 'universal' donors should be reserved for group O recipients only, or the blood used as packed red cells.

Rhesus System

This is a very complex system. At its simplest, it is convenient to classify individuals as *Rh positive* (85%) or *Rh negative* (15%) depending on the presence of the D antigen. This is largely a preventive measure to avoid transfusing a Rh negative recipient with the D antigen, which is the most immunogenic red-cell antigen after A and B.

At a more comprehensive level, it is convenient to consider the Rh system as a single gene complex on chromosome one, which gives rise to various combinations of three antigens C or c, D or d and E or e. These antigens are defined by corresponding antisera, with the exception of 'anti-d', which does not exist because d is thought to be amorphic. The gene complex is named either by the component antigens (e.g. CDe, cde) or by a single shorthand symbol (e.g. $R_1 = CDe$; $r = cde$). Thus, a person may inherit CDe (R_1) from one parent and cde (r) from the other, and have the genotype CDe/cde or R_1r.

Rhesus antigens are restricted to red cells and Rh antibodies are due to alloimmunisation by previous transfusion or pregnancy. They are usually IgG (sometimes with an IgM component), react best at 37°C, and do not fix complement. Haemolysis, when it occurs, is therefore extravascular and predominantly in the spleen (p. 35). Anti-D is the most important clinically; it has caused fatal haemolytic transfusion reactions and, until the recent success of anti-D prophylaxis, used to be a common cause of fetal death resulting from haemolytic disease of the newborn (HDN). The other Rh antibodies, although much less common, may nevertheless cause haemolytic transfusion reactions and HDN.

Other Blood Group Systems

Routine Rh(D) typing before blood transfusion and the success of anti-D prophylaxis for Rh(D) negative mothers bearing Rh(D) positive infants have greatly reduced the incidence of alloimmunisation to the D antigen. At the same time, the increasing use of blood transfusion has meant that more patients are being immunised by other antigens, especially Rh (c, E), Kell, Duffy, and Kidd. These antibodies have all been associated with haemolytic transfusion reactions and HDN.

DEMONSTRATION OF RED-CELL ANTIBODIES

The red cell is a convenient marker for antigens, and red-cell agglutination or lysis is a visible indication of antigen–antibody reaction. In the laboratory, various manipulations are necessary to promote agglutination of antibody-coated cells, depending on the Ig class of the antibody. The antibodies involved in immune haemolysis are IgM and IgG.

While IgM antibodies can agglutinate red cells suspended in saline, IgG antibodies are too small to bridge between the cells, which are kept apart by their negative surface charge. Other techniques are therefore required to promote agglutination of IgG antibody-coated cells, such as suspension in albumin or pretreatment with enzymes (e.g. papain), which probably assist agglutination by reducing the surface electrostatic charge keeping the cells apart.

The *antiglobulin (Coombs) test* is commonly used to demonstrate IgG antibody on red cells. The cells are thoroughly washed in normal saline to remove Ig not specifically bound to cell-surface antigens. The anti-human globulin (AHG) will bridge between antibody-coated cells and cause visible agglutination (Fig. 3.1). If monospecific antisera are used, it is possible to determine the Ig class and subclass of the antibody and to detect the presence of complement on the red cells. This provides useful information about the mechanism of haemolysis in the particular patient, and helps to establish the diagnosis.

The *direct* antiglobulin test is used to demonstrate *in vivo* attachment of antibodies to red cells, as in autoimmune haemolytic anaemia (p. 37) and allo-immune haemolytic disease of the newborn. When red cells are incubated *in vitro* with serum as the first step, and then tested with the AHG reagent, the procedure is called the *indirect* antiglobulin test. This has wide application in blood transfusion serology for red-cell antigen typing, antibody identification and compatibility testing.

PRE-TRANSFUSION COMPATIBILITY PROCEDURE

The aim of this procedure is to detect any significant antibodies in the patient's serum active against

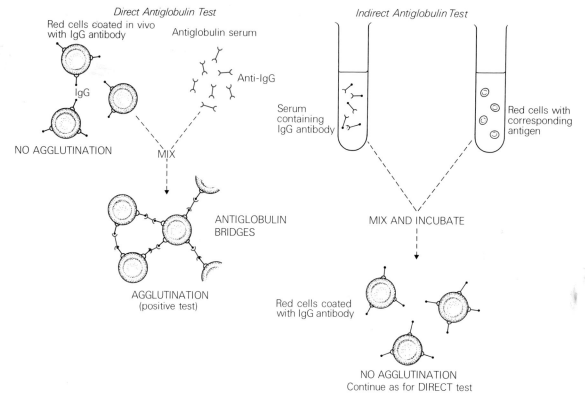

Fig. 3.1 *The direct and indirect anti-human globulin (Coombs) tests for demonstrating IgG antibodies. Similar reactions occur between complement components on the red cell (e.g. C3d) and corresponding anti-complement serum (anti-C3d).*

antigens on the donor's red cells. The following measures are taken to achieve donor–recipient compatibility.

ABO and RhD Grouping

Because of the natural occurrence of anti-A and anti-B, ABO compatibility is essential to avoid a haemolytic reaction. RhD typing, on the other hand, is primarily a preventive measure to avoid the high risk of alloimmunising an Rh(D) negative recipient with Rh(D) positive blood.

Antibody Screening

Anti-A and anti-B occur naturally and are detected as part of the ABO typing procedure. Other red-cell alloantibodies occur less regularly ('irregular' antibodies), and usually as a result of previous blood transfusions or pregnancy. It is becoming routine procedure to identify irregular antibodies in the recipient's serum before cross-matching, so that donor blood can be selected which lacks the corresponding antigens.

Selection of Donor Blood

Blood of the same ABO and RhD groups as the patient's is selected for cross-matching. It should also lack antigens corresponding to any irregular antibodies in the patient's serum.

Cross-Matching

In spite of antibody screening, it remains essential to do a direct cross-match of each donor's red cells against the patient's serum in order to confirm compatibility. In particular, this will detect any errors in labelling the donor units (e.g. exclude a potential ABO incompatibility). It will also reveal the presence in the patient's serum of a potentially haemolytic antibody against a low-incidence antigen which is not represented on the panel of screening cells but is present on the particular donor cells.

A combination of cross-matching tests is always used. This is necessary to detect both IgM and IgG antibodies as well as the complement component C3, which serves as a useful marker of antigen–antibody reaction, especially when antibody is present in undetectable amounts or has eluted from the cell in the testing procedure.

No matter how careful and comprehensive the laboratory techniques, it is essential to remember that the safety of blood transfusion depends on accurate patient and sample identification at all stages, starting with taking the blood sample from the patient for grouping and cross-matching and ending with the transfusion of compatible donor blood. Prevention of these 'clerical' errors would avoid most of the serious haemolytic transfusion reactions, almost all of which involve the ABO system.

CLINICAL CONSEQUENCES OF RED-CELL INCOMPATIBILITY

Donor–recipient compatibility is essential to ensure normal survival of the transfused cells and to avoid the harmful effects of a haemolytic transfusion reaction.

The clinical consequences of a haemolytic transfusion reaction are determined by:

a. the mechanism of haemolysis
b. the dose of antigen (i.e. the volume of red cells transfused)
c. the antibody concentration (or titre).

The mechanism of haemolysis depends on the Ig class of the antibody and its ability to activate complement. This also determines the site of haemolysis. *Intravascular haemolysis* is due to full activation of complement with consequent haemoglobinaemia and haemoglobinuria. This may be associated with IgM or IgG antibodies. *Extravascular haemolysis*, predominantly in the spleen, is a feature of IgG antibodies that do not fix complement. The antibody-coated red cells adhere to the sinusoidal macrophages of the spleen via specific receptors for the Fc part of IgG. The red cell is either phagocytosed or loses part of its membrane ('scission') and returns to the circulation as a microspherocyte. This is accompanied by some haemoglobinaemia, and the unconjugated bilirubin level is often raised. Haemolysis due to complement-fixing IgG antibodies may have both intra- and extra-vascular components.

The most dreaded complication of blood transfusion is severe intravascular haemolysis associated with ABO incompatibility. The clinical manifestations of severe haemolytic transfusion reactions are well recognised (Table 3.2), but fortunately not frequently encountered.

Table 3.2

Clinical   Manifestations   of   Severe   Intravascular   Haemolysis

---

Severe lumbar pain
Febrile rigors
Substernal tightness, dyspnoea
Persistent hypotension*
Urticaria
Vomiting, diarrhoea
Haemoglobinuria
Oozing from surgical wounds and needle punctures*
Renal shutdown
Jaundice

---

* Warning signs in anaesthetised patients

It is currently believed that the entire syndrome is due to the initial antigen–antibody reaction triggering a series of interactions between the complement and coagulation cascades. This results in the release of anaphylatoxins and vasoactive substances and in the initiation of disseminated intravascular coagulation (DIC). Acute renal failure appears to follow impaired renal blood flow and the deposition of fibrin thrombi in the small vessels.

An immediate haemolytic transfusion reaction is an acute emergency, and prompt diagnosis and treatment may be life-saving. At the first suspicion of a transfusion reaction, stop the transfusion (but maintain the drip for further use), because the severity of the reaction depends, among other factors, on the size of the dose of red-cell antigen. Diagnosis depends on demonstrating haemolysis in the patient and incompatibility between donor and recipient (Table 3.3). Emergency treatment of a severe haemolytic transfusion reaction aims to maintain the blood pressure and adequate renal perfusion. Consult a specialist renal physician as soon as possible. If the patient is anaemic, transfuse red

---

Table 3.3

Investigation of a Haemolytic Transfusion Reaction

Evidence of haemolysis
    Examine patient's plasma and urine for
    haemoglobin and its derivatives
    Blood film may show spherocytosis

Evidence of incompatibility
    Clerical checks. An identification error
    will indicate the type of incompatibility.
    If no evidence of clerical error, proceed
    as follows:
        Repeat ABO and RhD groups of patient and
        donor unit and screen for antibodies.
        Use patient's pre- and post-transfusion
        samples
        Repeat compatibility tests, using
        patient's pre- and post-transfusion
        serum
        Direct antiglobulin test on
        post-transfusion red cells may indicate
        antibody and/or complement

Evidence of bacterial infection of donor blood
    Gram stain and culture donor blood

---

cells compatible with the patient's serum. If the patient is bleeding, carry out laboratory tests for DIC and treat accordingly (p. 64).

Extravascular haemolysis (e.g. due to Rh antibodies) is not associated with the acute symptoms that characterise the transfusion of ABO incompatible blood. The rate of haemolysis is slower and the antibodies do not activate complement. However, immune extravascular haemolysis is associated with fever, sometimes with rigors, and there is variable anaemia and hyperbilirubinaemia.

A delayed haemolytic transfusion reaction may present some diagnostic confusion. This occurs when a patient, who has been alloimmunised by a previous transfusion or pregnancy, has no detectable antibodies at the time of cross-matching, but develops a secondary immune response to transfused red cells carrying the appropriate antigen. If enough antibody and donor red cells are present simultaneously, there will be a delayed haemolytic transfusion reaction (usually after 7–10 days). This may resemble an autoimmune haemolytic process, with a positive direct antiglobulin test (in this case due to alloantibody on the donor red cells), variable anaemia, reticulocytosis, spherocytosis and hyperbilirubinaemia. However, the preceding transfusion should suggest the correct diagnosis, and once this is made there is usually no need to do anything further as the process is self-limiting. Many of these delayed haemolytic reactions go unnoticed because they are less dramatic in presentation than the more immediate haemolytic reactions.

LEUCOCYTE AND PLATELET ANTIGENS

Leucocyte and platelet antigens may be exclusive to each cell type (cell-specific) or shared with other cells. Both platelet-specific and granulocyte-specific antigens are associated with significant clinical problems (p. 52). Of the shared antigens, the most important is the HLA (human leucocyte antigen) system, which has variable expression on the surface of most body cells. It is also called the major histocompatibility complex (MHC), which reflects the importance of HLA antigens in relation to transplantation.

HLA System

This system has four closely-linked loci, HLA-A, -B, -C and -D, coded by genes clustered together on the short arm of chromosome six. Each locus has many alleles, giving rise to many millions of different genotypes. Against such odds, the best chance of finding an HLA match lies within the family. One HLA gene complex (haplotype) is inherited from each parent *en bloc*, as crossing-over between the loci is uncommon. Since each parent has two haplotypes, there are four possible genotypes among the offspring, giving a one-in-four chance of two siblings being identical for the whole HLA complex.

HLA-A, -B and -C antigens are present on most cells, though generally absent from red cells, whereas HLA-D antigens have a more restricted distribution, being present mainly on B lymphocytes, monocytes, and some endothelial cells.

HLA antibodies are induced by pregnancy, transfusion or tissue grafting. As HLA antigens are best represented on lymphocytes, these cells are used for HLA typing and antibody identification. In the presence of complement, HLA antibodies will cause lysis of lymphocytes carrying the corresponding antigens in the lymphocytotoxicity test. This applies to HLA-A, -B

and -C antigens, whereas the HLA-D antigen is recognised by its ability to stimulate allogeneic T lymphocytes to divide in mixed lymphocyte cultures (MLC). Recently, by serological methods, an antigen has been defined on B-lymphocytes which is closely related to or identical with the HLA-D antigen; it has been designated HLA-DR (D-related).

The main application of HLA typing is to select compatible donor recipient pairs for renal and bone-marrow transplantation. It is also of value in selecting compatible platelet donors for patients who are refractory to platelet transfusions from random donors (p. 47). Another clinical interest in HLA typing is the association of some HLA antigens with certain diseases (e.g. HLA-B27 with ankylosing spondylitis), and over 100 diseases have been shown to have HLA associations. Just how HLA genes relate to disease susceptibility or resistance is uncertain.

DEMONSTRATION OF LEUCOCYTE AND PLATELET ANTIBODIES

Unlike red cells, leucocytes and platelets are difficult cells to work with serologically. The many and varied techniques that have been used for demonstrating antibodies to these cells bear witness to this. As a result, only a few acceptable procedures are in common use, and these are usually centralised in specialist laboratories.

HLA antigens are best represented on lymphocytes, and the lymphocytotoxicity test is most commonly used to detect HLA antibodies. A modified antihuman globulin technique, using fluorescent-labelled anti-human globulin to visualise the antigen–antibody reaction on the cell surface, is particularly suitable for demonstrating platelet, granulocyte and lymphocyte antibodies. This method detects both cell-specific antibodies and HLA antibodies.

CLINICAL CONSEQUENCES OF LEUCOCYTE AND PLATELET ANTIBODIES

Alloimmunisation to leucocyte and platelet antigens is most commonly due to transfusion or pregnancy, and the incidence of immunisation increases with the number of transfusions or pregnancies. The associated clinical problems depend on the specificity of the antibody, which determines the target cell involved. This has practical implications for transfusion, tissue transplantation, and neonatal immunohaematology.

Febrile transfusion reactions due to leucocyte antibodies are a common problem in multi-transfused patients. A typical reaction begins about $\frac{1}{2}$–2 hours after starting transfusion, when the patient feels cold and may have a rigor. This is associated with a rapid pulse and an abrupt rise in temperature. The reaction may last for up to 24 hours. In more severe reactions there may be anaphylactic effects due to complement activation, and sometimes severe dyspnoea. The granulocyte is the main target cell in these reactions, and granulocyte-specific antibodies seem to cause more severe reactions than HLA antibodies reacting with granulocytes. The severity of the reaction is increased by a high antibody concentration in the recipient's plasma and large numbers of leucocytes in the donor blood, the latter being accentuated by a rapid rate of transfusion. Short of cross-matching donor granulocytes, which is not a practical proposition (except of course in the case of granulocyte transfusions), febrile rigors can be prevented in alloimmunised recipients by using leucocyte-poor red cells.

Consequences other than febrile transfusion reactions may be summarised as follows:

a. *HLA-antibodies:*
Decreased survival of transfused
   i. platelets
   ii. granulocytes
Rejection of organ grafts
(not discussed in this chapter)

b. *Platelet-specific antibodies:*
Decreased survival of transfused platelets
Alloimmune neonatal thrombocytopenia

c. *Granulocyte-specific antibodies*
Decreased survival of transfused granulocytes
Alloimmune neonatal neutropenia

BLOOD COMPONENT THERAPY

Modern transfusion therapy is blood component therapy. The objectives are:

a. To give the patient the particular component he lacks, e.g. red cells, platelets, Factor VIII.
b. To substitute a normal for an abnormal component, e.g. whole-blood exchange for HDN; red-cell exchange for sickle cell disease; therapeutic plasmapheresis to remove abnormal proteins, antibodies or immune complexes.

In terms of blood resources, component therapy is more economical than the use of whole blood, as one donation may benefit more than one patient. Furthermore, the various fractions are more concentrated, and each can be stored under optimal conditions to ensure maximum therapeutic effect.

Whole Blood

Whole blood is usually reserved for treating acute blood loss, where both volume replacement and oxygen-carrying capacity are required, as in trauma, surgery, or severe haemorrhage from other causes. Even in this situation, plasma volume expanders and packed red cells can be used.

Packed Red Cells

A consequence of blood component therapy is the increasing use of plasma-reduced blood (packed red cells). This is the preparation of choice for an anaemic patient. Packed red cells have the same oxygen-carrying capacity as whole blood, but the volume is smaller, so minimising the risk of circulatory overload and cardiovascular failure.

Transfusion of an anaemic patient requires careful clinical judgement. It should not replace haematinic therapy, but should be reserved for the refractory anaemic patient who is unable to adapt to the lower oxygen-carrying capacity of the blood (e.g. by showing signs of incipient cardiovascular failure). (See also Circulatory Overload, and Transfusion Iron Overload)

Leucocyte-Poor Red Cells

Leucocyte-poor red cells are used to prevent febrile reactions in patients alloimmunised to leucocyte antigens (p. 45). They may also be used when it is desirable to minimise alloimmunisation of patients requiring repeated red-cell transfusions (e.g. thalassaemic children) or when there is a possibility of subsequent tissue transplantation.

Frozen Red Cells

Red cells containing a cryoprotective agent, such as glycerol, can be stored at low temperatures in liquid nitrogen for years. Prior to transfusion, the red cells are thawed and deglycerolised by washing. Frozen-washed red cells have the least leucocyte–platelet contamination of any preparation currently available, but cost limits their widespread use for this purpose. The process also effectively eliminates any hepatitis virus that may be present.

Special applications include storage of autologous red cells for subsequent transfusion, stockpiling selected blood groups for emergency and strategic purposes, and 'banking' red cells of special and rare blood groups.

Platelets

Platelet concentrates are prepared either by centrifugation of fresh whole blood units (six concentrates being the usual adult dose) or by plateletpheresis of a single donor. Pending improvements in methods for prolonged storage, platelets for transfusion should be as fresh as possible for maximum effect.

Platelet transfusions are used mainly to stop thrombocytopenic bleeding or to prevent bleeding, especially cerebral haemorrhage, in profoundly thrombocytopenic patients (i.e. platelet count $< 20 \times 10^9$/l). There are two situations to be considered: patients requiring platelet transfusion for a single, usually self-limiting incident, and those requiring longer-term platelet support (Table 3.4). Platelet transfusions are also used to stop bleeding or provide surgical cover in patients with platelet dysfunction. However, they are of little value in autoimmune thrombocytopenia (except perhaps for providing surgical cover, e.g. splenectomy for ITP), as the autoantibody cross-reacts with the transfused platelets, leading to their rapid clearance.

Understanding of the serology of platelet transfusion

Table 3.4

Indications for Platelet Transfusion

Thrombocytopenia ± bleeding
(i.e. therapeutic and prophylactic use)
  Limited cover for a single incident
    Surgical procedures
    'Washout' thrombocytopenia
      (massive transfusions of stored blood)
    Cardiac bypass thrombocytopenia
      (moderate thrombocytopenia ± dysfunction)
    Acute disseminated intravascular coagulation
      (usually give FFP ± platelets)
    Drug-induced immune thrombocytopenia
      (usually sufficient to stop drug)
  Longer-term platelet support of marrow-suppressed patients
    Intensive chemotherapy
      (e.g. remission induction in AML)
    Aplastic anaemia
Platelet dysfunction ± bleeding
  To stop bleeding or spontaneous bruising
  To provide surgical cover

is improving. The Rh(D) antigen is not represented in platelets and, although ABO antigens are present, ABO incompatibility is relatively unimportant for platelet survival. However, because of the variable, and sometimes heavy, red-cell contamination of platelet concentrates, it is usual practice to give platelets from ABO/Rh(D) compatible donors. The most important antigens in terms of platelet survival are the HLA (excluding HLA-D which is not represented on platelets) and platelet-specific systems. Alloimmunisation to these antigens may be a significant limiting factor in the supportive care of patients requiring repeated platelet transfusions. The selection of HLA-matched donors, however, will usually restore satisfactory post-transfusion platelet increments in alloimmunised patients.

Granulocytes

Granulocyte transfusion is still an experimental therapeutic procedure; it is rarely needed except in a few situations where antibiotics fail to control life-threatening infections associated with severe neutropenia ($< 0.5 \times 10^9$/l) due to marrow suppression. Success depends to a large extent on giving an adequate dose of granulocytes ($> 1.5 \times 10^{10}$/day). Transfusion should be continued for several days.

Leucapheresis is essential for the collection of enough granulocytes from a single normal donor for an effective transfusion. Patients with chronic granulocytic leukaemia are sometimes used as donors because of their high circulating granulocyte count.

Because of the heavy red-cell contamination of granulocyte concentrates, it is necessary to select ABO- and RhD-compatible donors, and to carry out a red-cell cross-match before transfusion. Repeated granulocyte transfusions from random donors lead to alloimmunisation to HLA and granulocyte-specific antigens. These antibodies shorten the survival of the transfused cells and also impair their phagocytic function. Furthermore, febrile transfusion reactions and more severe complications due to pulmonary leuco-stasis may curtail the use of granulocyte transfusions.

Plasma Components

Details of the plasma components available for clinical use are summarised in Table 3.5.

Table 3.5

Plasma Components for Clinical Use

Component	Contents	Indications for use	Hepatitis risk (a)
Plasma protein fraction (PPF)	4–5% albumin in buffered saline	Blood volume expansion Plasma replacement (e.g. burns, therapeutic plasmapheresis)	0
Human albumin	Salt-poor albumin 25% solution	Albumin replacement in acute hypoalbuminaemia, often with diuretics	0
Fresh frozen plasma (FFP) (b)	Plasma + all clotting factors (including labile factors V & VIII)	Multiple clotting factor deficiencies, e.g. DIC; massive transfusion of stored blood; warfarin overdose; liver disease	1
Cryoprecipitate (b)	Factor VIII von Willebrand factor Fibrinogen	Haemophilia von Willebrand's disease Fibrinogen deficiency	1
Factor VIII concentrate	Factor VIII	Haemophilia	2
Factor IX concentrate	Factor IX Also, II, X ± VII	Christmas disease	2
Human normal Ig	γ-globulin	Hypogammaglobulinaemia Prophylaxis of common viral diseases	0
Human specific Ig	Specific antibodies from convalescent serum or hyperimmunised donors	Rh anti-D Tetanus, herpes zoster etc. for prophylaxis or disease attenuation	0

(a) 0 = no risk (preparation eliminates virus)
    1 = same as whole blood
    2 = greater than whole blood (pooled preparations)
(b) ABO compatibility essential

ADVERSE EFFECTS OF TRANSFUSION

The unwanted effects of transfusion may be classified as below.

Immunological Consequences

These have already been discussed, and may be summarised as follows:

a. Alloimmunisation
   Red cell, leucocyte and platelet antigens
   Plasma protein antigens
b. Incompatibility
   Haemolytic transfusion reaction
   Intravascular haemolysis
      ABO incompatibility
   Extravascular haemolysis
      Immediate
      Delayed
   Leucocyte and platelet antibodies
   Febrile rigors (granulocytes)
   Post-transfusion purpura (platelets)
   Poor survival of transfused platelets and granulocytes
   Plasma protein antibodies
   Urticarial and anaphylactic reactions
   (severe reactions associated with anti-IgA antibodies)

Metabolic Disturbances

Stored blood is cold (4°C), acid (pH 6.6–6.8), and contains citrate anticoagulant, high levels of potassium (leaked from red cells), ammonia (from adenosine), and reduced red-cell 2,3-DPG (p. 4). This is usually not a problem, but the transfusion of large volumes of cold stored blood may lead to cardiac and metabolic disturbances, e.g. ventricular fibrillation, metabolic acidosis.

Haemostatic Defects

Stored blood is deficient in platelets and labile clotting factors (V and VIII). Therefore, massive transfusion of stored blood will cause a dilution of labile clotting factors and moderate thrombocytopenia (40–70 × 10^9/l). It is common practice to give two units of FFP with every 8–10 units of stored blood to replace the depleted labile clotting factors. The moderate thrombocytopenia usually does not require platelet transfusion.

Microaggregates in Stored Blood

Microaggregates of platelets, leucocytes and fibrin are formed in stored blood. It is uncertain to what extent they cause pulmonary microvascular obstruction, but it is a safe policy to use special microaggregate filters when more than five units of stored blood are to be given rapidly.

Circulatory Overload

This complication arises most commonly in patients with severe and long-standing anaemia. It is essential to resist the temptation to transfuse newly-diagnosed patients with severe uncomplicated megaloblastic or iron deficiency anaemia. Such patients are usually in cardiorespiratory equilibrium and can afford to await the effective results of specific haematinics. If it is considered necessary to transfuse such a patient, packed red cells should be given very slowly (with or without diuretic therapy), or an exchange transfusion may be indicated.

Transfusion Iron Overload (Haemosiderosis)

Repeated red-cell transfusion over many years, in the absence of blood loss, causes deposition of iron in the reticuloendothelial tissue at the rate of 200–250 mg per unit of blood. After about 100 units, the liver, myocardium and endocrine glands are damaged. This is a major problem in children with thalassaemia major and other patients with chronic refractory anaemias. Iron chelation therapy with desferrioxamine is commonly used to reduce iron overload in this situation.

Disease Transmission

The most frequent serious complication of blood transfusion therapy is viral hepatitis.

All blood donations are screened for hepatitis B surface antigen HB_sAg (Australia antigen), the incidence of positive results among first-time donors being about 0.1%. In spite of this, post-transfusion hepatitis remains a problem, due mainly to non-A non-B hepatitis, for which there are no suitable screening tests. The risk of infection is highest with pooled blood products, e.g. Factor VIII concentrate for haemophilia (Table 3.5), and in chronically transfused patients.

Other infections transmitted by blood transfusion include syphilis, for which all donors are screened, and malaria, which is a potential risk in donors who have visited or lived in areas where malaria is endemic.

Infected Blood

Bacterial contamination of donor blood is very rare, but may cause profound shock soon after starting the transfusion. This must be differentiated from an acute intravascular haemolytic reaction. Gram-negative bacilli capable of growing at 4°C are the most common cause. Shock should be treated vigorously with supportive measures, and antibiotics should be given as soon as possible.

FETO-MATERNAL INCOMPATIBILITY WITH RESPECT TO BLOOD-CELL ANTIGENS

Pregnancy is a special situation where fetal blood cells cross the placenta and may immunise the mother against antigens inherited from the father. Alloimmunisation *per se* has no harmful effect on the mother, but it predisposes her to possible immunological complications from a subsequent blood transfusion or tissue transplantation. However, maternal IgG antibodies so formed are actively transported across the placenta into the fetal circulation. The clinical effects depend on the specificity of the antibody. Although HLA antibodies are often formed during pregnancy, they do not appear to cause any harm to the fetus. Each cell-specific antibody, on the other hand, causes a characteristic disease. Red-cell specific antibodies cause haemolytic disease of the newborn. Platelet-specific antibodies cause alloimmune neonatal thrombocytopenia. Granulocyte-specific antibodies cause alloimmune neonatal neutropenia.

Haemolytic Disease of the Newborn (HDN)

HDN is a form of haemolytic anaemia affecting the fetus and newborn infant. It occurs when maternal alloantibody to fetal red-cell antigens crosses the placenta and causes haemolysis of fetal red cells. As IgG is the only immunoglobulin transferred across the placenta, only red-cell antibodies of this class cause HDN.

Rhesus HDN

Anti-D causes the most severe form of HDN. Today, we can effectively eliminate the disease by preventing the mother from becoming alloimmunised against the RhD antigen. It should be emphasised that routine RhD typing prevents alloimmunisation by blood transfusion.

Maternal alloimmunisation

This may occur when an Rh-negative (dd) mother has an Rh(D)-positive fetus. When the placenta separates at delivery, fetal red cells enter the maternal circulation. The risk of Rh(D) immunisation depends on the maternal dose of fetal red cells and the mother's ability to respond to the antigenic stimulus; approximately 30% of individuals are 'non-responders' in this respect. Furthermore, ABO incompatibility between mother and fetus effectively protects the Rh-negative mother against immunisation by the fetal Rh(D) antigen. The overall risk of Rh immunisation is about 15% if the fetus is ABO-compatible. The precise mechanism of the protection afforded by ABO incompatibility is not clear, but it is thought to be related to rapid clearance of ABO-incompatible fetal red cells, so that the mother is not immunised by the D antigen which they also carry. Similarly, the administration of anti-D immunoglobulin to an Rh(D)-negative individual, at the same time as a dose of Rh(D)-positive red cells, will suppress primary immunisation. The practical application of this has led to the virtual prevention of anti-D HDN.

Prevention of maternal alloimmunisation

It is standard antenatal care to determine the ABO and Rh(D) groups of all mothers and screen the serum for antibodies. Anti-D is now administered to every Rh(D)-negative mother giving birth to an Rh(D)-positive child, provided she is not already immunised to the D antigen by a previous pregnancy or blood transfusion. It is essential that the dose of anti-D given should be adequate to clear all the fetal red cells from the maternal circulation. The dose of anti-D is determined by the Kleihauer test, which estimates the number of fetal cells in the maternal blood. A blood film of maternal blood is made soon after delivery. Since adult, but not fetal, haemoglobin is eluted at acid pH, the fetal red cells contrast with the maternal red-cell ghosts. From this, an estimate of the transplacental bleed can be made. The appropriate dose of anti-D should be given as soon as possible after delivery and not later than 72 hours *post partum*.

In cases of abortion, it is assumed that the fetus is Rh(D) positive (unless the father is also Rh negative), and anti-D should be given. Any event during pregnancy which might lead to a transplacental bleed (e.g. trauma, obstetric manipulations, amniocentesis, fetoscopy) should be covered by an appropriate injection of anti-D, determined by a Kleihauer test.

Fetal consequences of maternal alloimmunisation

Once sensitised to the D antigen, whether by a previous pregnancy or blood transfusion, an Rh-negative mother will have an anamnestic response during the next Rh(D)-positive pregnancy. The worst prognosis for the fetus is associated with high maternal levels of anti-D from an early stage of pregnancy. Intensive plasmapheresis to reduce the maternal anti-D level has been successful in reducing the severity of the disease in such cases.

Maternal antibody crosses the placenta and haemolyses fetal red cells. The severity of haemolysis is assessed by measuring changes in the bilirubin content of amniotic fluid, which is obtained by amniocentesis. In severe disease there is intrauterine fetal death associated with severe anaemia, enlarged liver, spleen and heart, and severe generalised oedema (hydrops fetalis). Some severely affected fetuses can be rescued by intrauterine transfusions until it is safe to interrupt pregnancy. On the other hand, some fetuses have severe, but well compensated, haemolysis and do not need intrauterine transfusion. Excess bilirubin produced *in utero* is transferred across the placenta and excreted by the maternal liver. On delivery, however, the premature liver is unable to conjugate bilirubin, which rapidly accumulates because of the continuing haemolysis, and there is a risk of brain-stem damage (kernicterus).

Tests on cord blood at birth show variable anaemia, nucleated red cells, a high reticulocyte count, and raised serum bilirubin. The red cells group as Rh(D)-positive, and the direct antiglobulin test is positive. These babies usually need repeated exchange transfusions to correct the anaemia and reduce the high levels of unconjugated bilirubin.

The mildest form of the disease occurs when the mother has very little antibody or an antibody which reacts only weakly with the fetal red cells. At birth the cord cells are antibody-coated (positive direct antiglobulin test), but there is little or no evidence of haemolysis and no treatment is required. This is the commonest form of the disease, accounting for about half of affected infants.

HDN due to Other Antibodies

The success of anti-D prophylaxis has reduced the number of cases of HDN due to anti-D, and consequently the relative proportion of cases due to other antibodies has increased. The commonest other causes of HDN are anti-c, anti-E and anti-K (Kell), but almost every other red-cell IgG antibody has been reported as a cause of HDN.

ABO-HDN

This is considered separately, as a number of special factors combine to protect the fetus from the effects of ABO incompatibility. For practical purposes, only group O individuals make IgG anti-A and anti-B. Therefore, only A or B infants of group O mothers are at risk from ABO-HDN. Although 25% of births are susceptible, only about 1% are affected; even then the condition is usually mild and very rarely severe enough to need exchange transfusion (about 1 in 3 000). Two mechanisms protect the fetus against anti-A and anti-B; one is the relative weakness of A and B antigens at birth, and the other is the widespread distribution of A and B glycoproteins in body fluids and tissues, which diverts much of the IgG antibody that crosses the placenta away from the red-cell 'target'.

ABO-HDN may be seen in the first incompatible pregnancy, because the group O primigravida has already made IgG anti-A and anti-B in response to various immunising stimuli. This is unlike anti-D HDN, where immunisation usually takes place at the end of the first pregnancy, the first child being unaffected.

There is as yet no satisfactory test to determine which mothers are likely to have an affected child. At birth, ABO-HDN is suspected if a group O mother has an A or B child who is jaundiced. The direct antiglobulin test usually demonstrates IgG on cord red cells, which can be eluted and shown to have anti-A or anti-B specificity. Other red-cell antibodies must be excluded, as well as other causes of neonatal jaundice. The degree of haemolysis is usually mild and most babies require no treatment. The blood film of an affected child characteristically shows spherocytosis and reticulocytosis, and there may also be nucleated red cells.

Alloimmune Neonatal Thrombocytopenia and Neutropenia

These conditions, which are relatively uncommon, are due to immunisation of the mother against fetal platelet- and granulocyte-specific antigens inherited from the father. The high frequency of first-pregnancy immunisation suggests that leucocytes and platelets invade the maternal circulation at a much earlier stage than red cells.

Diagnosis depends on demonstrating a cell-specific alloantibody in the maternal and fetal serum that reacts with the baby's platelets or granulocytes. At the time of diagnosis, the baby's cells are often not available in adequate numbers for testing, and so the father's cells, which carry the relevant antigen, are a more convenient alternative.

Neonatal thrombocytopenia may also be due to placental transfer of IgG platelet autoantibodies from mothers with autoimmune thrombocytopenia.

4

Haemostasis

INTRODUCTION

The prevention or arrest of haemorrhage (haemostasis) is one of the body's fundamental homeostatic mechanisms. Platelet function, vessel contraction and blood coagulation protect the body by reducing blood loss, and fibrinolysis ensures vessel patency. Failure of any component of these complex systems results in excess bleeding. This can vary from leakage of a few red cells from capillaries to the more dramatic haemorrhage seen in severe haemophilia, thrombocytopenia, or consumption coagulopathy in which the patient may bleed spontaneously from a multitude of sites and eventually die of uncontrollable haemorrhage. It is convenient for descriptive purposes to consider these conditions separately, but the reactions involved are intimately interlinked and are also associated with other triggered enzyme systems in plasma, such as the kallikrein–kinin system, complement activation, and the generation of permeability factors.

NORMAL HAEMOSTASIS

Platelet Function

When a blood vessel is cut, the result is adhesion of a single layer of platelets to the exposed subendothelial collagen, basement membrane and elastic fibres. Adhesion causes the platelets to release the constituents of their granules, particularly amines such as adenosine diphosphate (ADP), adenosine triphosphate (ATP), and the vasoactive material, serotonin (5-hydroxytryptamine: 5-HT). These amines are liberated into the immediate environment of the adherent platelet and rapidly cause neighbouring platelets to change from disc shapes to spheroid forms with pseudopodia. These altered platelets aggregate together and form a mass with the already adherent platelets which plugs the defect in the vessel. This reaction is rapid and occurs within a few seconds of vessel injury (Fig. 4.1a).

In addition to the above mechanism, platelet membrane phospholipase is activated during aggregation and this releases arachidonic acid from platelet phospholipid (Fig. 4.2). The arachidonic acid is acted on by cyclo-oxygenase, converting it to unstable prostaglandin endoperoxides which are then converted to thromboxane A_2 (TXA_2), a powerful platelet-aggregating agent that enhances the rapid accumulation of platelets at the site of vessel injury. In addition, TXA_2 is a powerful vasoconstrictor.

Local platelet activation stimulates a similar parallel series of reactions in the vascular intima, during which endoperoxides are converted to prostacyclin that acts in an opposing way, inhibiting platelet aggregation (Fig. 4.2). In due course, a balance is established between the production of TXA_2 by platelets and prostacyclin by vascular endothelium.

Collagen simultaneously absorbs plasma factor XII and activates the coagulation pathway by a series of rather slow reactions which result in thrombin and fibrin generation (Figs. 4.1b and 4.3). Thrombin is also a powerful platelet-aggregating agent. Thus, at least three separate mechanisms act synchronously and synergistically to produce platelet aggregation at the site of injury: amine release (ADP and 5-HT), thromb-

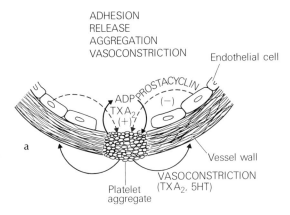

ADHESION
RELEASE
AGGREGATION
VASOCONSTRICTION

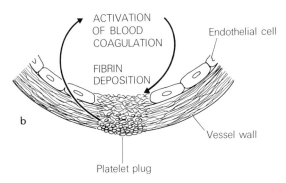

Fig. 4.1 *Platelet plug formation (a) and stabilisation of the platelet plug by fibrin formation (b).*

oxane A_2 generation, and thrombin formation by the coagulation mechanism.

At the same time as the above events, a phospholipid becomes available on the platelet surface (platelet factor 3, PF_3), and this plays a key role in promoting the blood coagulation pathway (Fig. 4.3). It is not released into the plasma but acts as a surface onto which coagulation factors bind and then react as a result of physical proximity.

Serotonin (5-HT) is also liberated by adherent and aggregated platelets and has a powerful vasoconstrictive function. Together with TXA_2, it causes vessel constriction and reduced blood flow at the site of formation of the platelet aggregate and prevents it from being washed away by the force of blood flow. The platelet aggregate stabilises as fibrin is formed in and around the aggregated platelets (Fig. 4.1b).

Thus haemostasis is initially dependent on platelet and vessel function, which together result in formation of a platelet plug. At this early stage coagulation seems to play little part but, if there is a deficiency of clotting factors (such as in haemophilia), excess bleeding occurs later on as a result of failure in fibrin generation and hence failure to stabilise the platelet plug. Such a situation is seen in clinical practice if a haemophilic patient has a tooth extracted without any factor VIII replacement. Initial haemostasis is normal, there is no bleeding, and the patient returns home. Excess bleeding begins only when the platelet plug, which has not been stabilised by formation of fibrin, is washed away as the vasoconstrictor effect of 5-HT and TXA_2 declines.

Vascular Structure and Function

There is clear evidence from clinical studies that normality of the endothelial cell lining, basement membrane, and supporting collagen and elastic fibres is essential for haemostasis.

Injury to an arteriole or venule leads to immediate contraction of the muscle layer and vasoconstriction, as a result of reflex autonomic action as well as of the serotonin–TXA_2-mediated mechanisms already described. This response is transient and wears off over a period of 10–20 minutes. No such muscular mechanism exists in capillaries, but flow into a capillary bed is controlled by a 'precapillary sphincter' which may serve the same function. In addition, there is evidence from experimental work that occlusion of capillaries may be a result of endothelial adhesion. This period of vasoconstriction allows time for platelet and fibrin deposition to occur and thereby secure haemostasis.

The normal capillary is a simple structure consisting of a tube lined with endothelial cells on a basement membrane supported by pericytes and collagen fibres. The endothelial lining of the vascular tree consists of a single layer of deformable cells, with their long axes aligned to the direction of blood flow. The cells are joined together by intercellular bridges and are coated by a thin layer of mucopolysaccharide which extends into the potential space between cells. This continuous sheet of cells retains blood within the vascular tree, stops platelets and fibrin forming in excess, but still allows the passage of gases, nutrients and fluids into the tissues of the body. The endothelial cells produce prostacyclin, factor VIII-related antigen (VIII:RAg), and a fibrinolytic activator. Prostacyclin is the main meta-

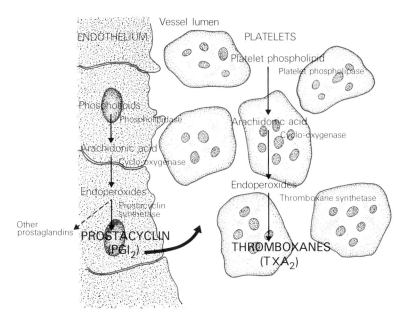

Fig. 4.2 *Platelet–vessel wall interaction after vascular damage. The aggregative effect of the thromboxane A$_2$ (TXA$_2$) produced by platelets is opposed by the prostacyclin (PGI$_2$) produced in the vascular endothelium.*

bolic product of arachidonic acid in vascular tissues (Fig. 4.2). In addition, prostacyclin causes already-formed platelet aggregates to disaggregate, and this may be a further protective function. The half-life of prostacyclin in the blood is about 2–3 minutes, implying that local stimulation of production has only a local effect.

There is also evidence that normal, circulating platelets are required to maintain the functional integrity of the endothelial layer. Atrophy of the endothelium follows when platelets are quantitatively or qualitatively deficient, and it therefore seems likely that they have a nutritional role.

Blood Coagulation

Contact of blood with exposed subendothelial collagen and elastic fibres initiates a complex series of reactions which result in the formation of fibrin. Blood clotting factors are present in the plasma as inert proenzymes (zymogens) which are converted to an active form (designated with the suffix a), and this in turn activates

the following zymogen. This triggered enzyme system, termed a 'cascade' or 'waterfall' sequence of reactions, is shown in Fig. 4.3.

The coagulation mechanism may best be described in distinct phases, although it should be appreciated that important feedback inhibition and accelerator mechanisms exist.

The contact phase of blood coagulation

Factors XII and XI are the major factors in this phase of the coagulation process.

Factor XII may be activated by a variety of artificial surfaces (e.g. glass, kaolin, dacron, nylon) as well as by collagen, basement membrane, uric acid crystals, endotoxin and the soaps of saturated fatty acids. Factor XIIa holds a central position in the initiation of other triggered enzyme reactions, e.g. kinin generation, complement activation, fibrinolysis and the generation of permeability factors, all of which have key roles in haemostasis.

It is a paradox that patients with factor XII deficiency have no clinical haemostatic defect, despite failure of

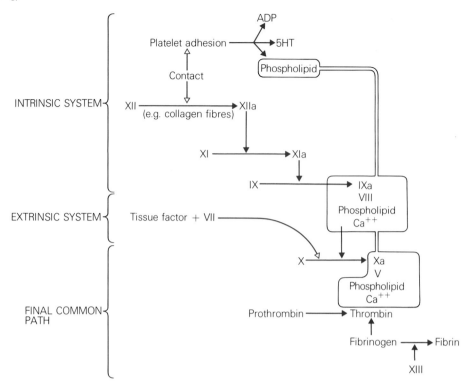

Fig. 4.3 *The coagulation cascade. A variety of inert precursors are present in plasma which, when stimulated, react sequentially. Two systems are present, intrinsic and extrinsic, having a final common path which leads to fibrin formation.*

their blood to clot in a glass test tube. This, presumably, shows that alternate pathways of clotting exist.

Activated factor XII (XIIa) activates factor XI. Deficiency of factor XI, which is uncommon, is transmitted in an autosomal recessive fashion and results in a tendency towards mild to moderate bleeding.

Formation of factor IXa

Activation of factor IX (Christmas factor) is a result of the enzymic action of factor XIa in the presence of calcium ions.

Factor IX is the factor which is deficient in patients with Christmas disease, a condition associated with life-long haemostatic difficulties with the same spectrum of clinical problems as haemophilia (see later).

Formation of factor Xa

There are two separate pathways for the generation of factor Xa. Both are necessary for normal haemostasis.

a. *The intrinsic pathway–slow factor Xa generation.* This step (Fig. 4.3) involves the interaction of factor IXa, phospholipid, calcium ions and factor VIII (antihaemophilic factor). The phospholipid, produced by the platelets, brings activated factor IX and factor VIII together to form a complex which converts factor X to Xa.

Factor VIII has distinct properties associated with different parts of the molecule. Factor VIIIc is of low molecular weight and has the procoagulant activity. This part of the molecule is deficient in patients with classic haemophilia and is also at a low level in patients with von Willebrand's disease. Factor VIII-related antigen (VIIIR:Ag) is that part of the molecule which is precipitated by rabbit antibodies to purified factor VIII. It has a very high molecular weight and acts as a carrier protein for factor VIIIc. It has been shown that, in classic haemophilia, a protein immunologically identical with normal factor VIII is produced, but this has no procoagulant activity. In von Willebrand's disease, factor VIIIR:Ag is reduced in amount and may have electrophoretic differences from normal VIIIR:Ag. When the antibiotic, ristocetin, is added to normal platelet-rich plasma, it induces platelet aggregation. This is mediated through part of the factor VIIIR:Ag molecule. In von Willebrand's disease this activity is diminished or absent, and the activity responsible is called factor VIIIR:WF. Factor VIIIR:Ag and VIIIR:WF are synthesised in endothelial cells and are closely related, the latter activity probably corresponding to a particular configuration of part of the VIIIR:Ag molecule.

b. *The extrinsic pathway—rapid factor Xa generation* (Fig. 4.3). This pathway requires the participation of a tissue factor (i.e. extrinsic to blood, and sometimes called thromboplastin), factor VII and calcium ions. These components form a complex, factor VII is activated in the process, and this in turn activates factor X.

The individual importance of these two mechanisms of factor X activation is not clear in normal haemostasis, but deficiencies of factor VII or X result in a moderate bleeding tendency.

Factors II, VII, IX and X are produced in the liver and contain γ-carboxyglutamate. The carboxylation of glutamate involves vitamin K. Oral anticoagulants inhibit this action of vitamin K, resulting in the formation of functionally inert proteins which have immunological identity with the active factor.

Formation of thrombin

The enzyme thrombin is formed by activation of the inert precursor, prothrombin (factor II), by a complex formed by factor Xa, factor V and phospholipid in the presence of ionic calcium.

Deficiency of factor V is a rare disorder and is characterised by a severe bleeding tendency.

In addition to converting fibrinogen (factor I) to fibrin, thrombin acts on platelets (to cause irreversible aggregation); it also alters the factor VIII molecule (accelerat-

ing the earlier stages of the system) and activates factor XIII (ensuring the stability of forming fibrin).

Formation of fibrin and its stabilisation

The conversion of fibrinogen to fibrin involves proteolysis, polymerisation and stabilisation. The enzyme, thrombin, cleaves the fibrinogen molecule at one end, producing small peptide fragments and larger fibrin monomers. Removal of the fibrinopeptides allows the fibrin monomers to link together spontaneously to form a fibrin polymer which is stabilised by cross-links catalysed by factor XIII, already activated by thrombin or by factor Xa.

Physiological Inhibitors of Blood Coagulation

It is probable that every activated coagulation factor in the cascade has one or more inhibitors which regulate the rate of generation of the active product or determine its destruction. The purpose of these would seem to be to limit the activation of clotting and to protect against inadvertent deposition of fibrin in the vascular tree.

The most important of these inhibitors is antithrombin III (At III). In patients with hereditary deficiency of At III, the low levels are associated with an increased tendency to thrombosis in veins and, rarely, in arteries, particularly in pregnancy. Depression of normal levels is caused by the use of oral contraceptives, and occurs in cirrhosis of the liver, in the nephrotic syndrome, and in conditions associated with disseminated intravascular coagulation.

Fibrinolysis

Fibrinolysis is the process by which fibrin formed in the circulation is enzymatically degraded into soluble products (fibrin degradation products – FDPs – Fig. 4.4). The purpose of this fibrinolytic process is to maintain patency in the vascular tree by controlling excess fibrin deposition on the vessel wall. The body appears to maintain a balance between fibrin deposition and its removal. There are four components in the system: plasminogen, plasmin, activators, and inhibitors.

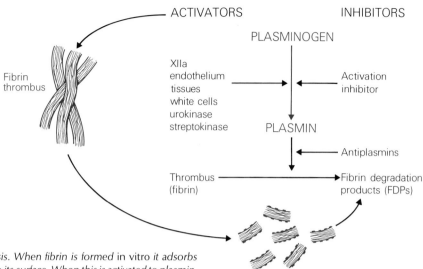

Fig. 4.4 *Fibrinolysis. When fibrin is formed* in vitro *it adsorbs plasminogen onto its surface. When this is activated to plasmin, it selectively digests the fibrin to produce low-molecular-weight products which are removed in the circulation. Due to the physical proximity of plasmin and fibrin, inhibitors in the surrounding plasma have no effect on the reaction, but they do inhibit its spread to other plasma factors.*

Plasminogen

This is the inert precursor of plasmin and, while present in most body fluids, has its highest concentration in plasma. Plasminogen has a high affinity for fibrin and is adsorbed to the thrombus as it forms. Reduced plasminogen levels may be due to excess consumption (in disseminated intravascular coagulation and during thrombolytic therapy), or to deficient production (in infancy and advanced hepatic cirrhosis). Higher levels than normal are found in patients after trauma, surgery, infection, thrombosis, and disseminated cancer.

Plasmin

Plasmin is the proteolytic enzyme formed from plasminogen. It is not normally detectable in human plasma because of the presence of an excess of inhibitors. The prime function of plasma is to digest fibrin, but it has a wide spectrum of activity against other plasma proteins such as fibrinogen and factors V and VIII. However, because of the physical association of plasminogen with the fibrin in a thrombus, plasmin formed by activation digests fibrin selectively to form low-molecular-weight breakdown products (FDPs).

Activators of fibrinolysis

Activators of plasminogen occur in most body tissues and fluids, including plasma, and are found also in the culture media of certain bacteria (e.g. streptococcus produces streptokinase).

It is not clear where the normal plasma activator is produced. At least three sources may be responsible:

a. *Venous endothelium.* This is a rich source of plasminogen activator, which is liberated in response to a variety of physiological stimuli (exercise, anoxia, stress, and catecholamines) or by infusion of pharmacologic agents (nicotinic acid or vasopressin analogues). The liberation of such an activator may be used to assess the total 'fibrinolytic potential' of a patient, and this has been shown to be deficient in patients with premature arterial disease. It may also be liberated in excess from extremely vascular tumours to produce a fibrinolytic defect in haemostasis.

b. *Factor XII-dependent activator.* Activation of factor XII to XIIa leads to the generation of a plasminogen activator. This activity is absent in patients with factor

XII deficiency, but they do not seem to have a tendency to thrombosis.

c. *Red-cell, white-cell and tissue activators.* Many cell types contain activators which are different in molecular weight. The activator urokinase, produced by renal cells, has been partially purified for therapeutic use. The role of activators in physiology is not clear but, in states such as leukaemia or acute haemolysis, excess production of red- or white-cell activators may produce a haemostatic abnormality. In addition to the activators found in blood, many other tissues contain activators. Their physiological role is local but, in situations such as severe trauma, surgery or malignancy, excess tissue activator may be produced in sufficient amounts to produce a severe systemic hyperplasminaemic state with resultant bleeding.

Inhibitors of fibrinolysis

At least six inhibitors of plasmin have been shown to exist in human plasma, but it seems likely that only two are of physiological importance. These are α_2-macroglobulin and α_2-antiplasmin. They act by forming complexes with plasmin, which is rendered enzymatically inactive thus ensuring containment of the fibrinolytic reaction.

ABNORMAL HAEMOSTASIS

Vascular Disorders

The clinical features of vascular abnormalities of haemostasis usually include a history of repeated epistaxis, spontaneous easy bruising, bleeding from the gums after brushing teeth, and bleeding from other mucosal surfaces, including the genito-urinary and gastrointestinal tracts. Examination of the skin may show petechial or purpuric spots (petechiae are pin-point capillary haemorrhages in the skin, while the term purpura refers to more extensive haemorrhage; ecchymoses are still larger sheet haemorrhages involving subcutaneous tissues).

Mechanical purpura

Perhaps the most common cause of purpura is a sudden rise in capillary pressure with resultant leakage of red cells. This may occur in normal people after taking the blood pressure, if the sphygmomanometer cuff pressure is raised above 200 mmHg. A rise in capillary pressure may also occur during breath-holding in attacks of whooping cough, in epileptic fits, and after prolonged vomiting.

In many cases, no pathological basis is ever found for easy bruising, particularly in women, and these lesions have been called 'devil's pinches' or purpura simplex.

Purpura with an 'allergic' basis

The basic mechanism is unknown but may involve destruction of endothelial cells and basement membrane by an immunological process. The diseases which are associated are rheumatoid arthritis, systemic lupus erythematosus, polyarteritis nodosa, Henoch–Schönlein syndrome and subacute bacterial endocarditis. Light microscopy shows evidence of perivascular cuffing with leucocytes, and electron-dense material (immune complexes) can be seen between and under the endothelial cells. This type of vasculitis may also be associated with a variety of drugs such as penicillins, isoniazid, aspirin, thiazide diuretics and oxytetracycline.

Microembolism and thrombosis

Purpura associated with disseminated intravascular coagulation, fat embolism, septicaemia, dysproteinaemia and very high white cell counts probably have a similar aetiology. It is not clear whether capillary occlusion or endothelial damage with subsequent thrombosis is the primary mechanism involved.

Hereditary haemorrhagic telangiectasia

This uncommon disorder, which is inherited in an autosomal dominant pattern, is characterised by localised dilatation of venules and capillaries throughout the body. The lesions (telangiectasia) are particularly common on the mucosa of the mouth and nose, and epistaxis is a common presenting symptom of the disorder. Bleeding, however, may occur at a variety of other sites including the gastrointestinal and respiratory tracts, and iron-deficiency anaemia may result. Treatment consists of local measures to stop bleeding, and iron or blood replacement.

Decreased strength of supporting structures

This is often seen in old people (senile purpura) and in patients on steroid therapy or with Cushing's syndrome. Sections of the skin show atrophy of the supporting connective tissue of capillaries. The repeated leakage of red cells, in association with diminished white cell function, leaves brownish areas of haemosiderin (age spots). There is also evidence that ageing collagen fibres are less effective in producing platelet adhesion.

The purpura of scurvy is due partly to failure of normal collagen synthesis and partly to a functional defect in platelets. In adults, clinical disease usually involves only a few skin petechiae, but in babies extensive haemorrhage may be seen in the subperiosteum.

Deficiency of capillary support is also found in a variety of genetic defects such as Marfan's syndrome, Ehlers–Danlos syndrome, osteogenesis imperfecta, and pseudoxanthoma elasticum. In these conditions there may be abnormalities of collagen, fibroblasts, or elastic fibres.

Infiltration of the perivascular tissues of the capillaries and small arterioles by amyloid may increase permeability and decrease strength of the vessel. The lesions are typically seen in the facial areas and not in the dependent parts of the body. The diagnosis is made by skin biopsy.

Platelet Disorders

The clinical manifestations of platelet abnormalities, which resemble those already described for the vascular disorders, are characterised by skin petechiae and mucosal bleeding.

Quantitative defects in platelets

A fall in the number of functioning platelets is associated with a tendency to bleed, and this is directly related to the absolute number of platelets. Haemo-stasis is usually intact until a platelet count of about $40 \times 10^9/l$ is reached. Administration of fresh platelets in this situation is known to be clinically effective; it would appear that they act directly on the endothelium, and haemostasis may be achieved without any rise in the measured platelet count. In patients with thrombocytopenia the endothelial cells themselves are also abnormal, being about half the thickness of normal endothelial cells. These changes in the endothelial cells can be altered by steroids, which produce haemostasis without any rise in the platelet count.

The causes of thrombocytopenia are multiple and are shown in Table 4.1. The thrombocytopenias caused by increased destruction, abnormal distribution, or dilutional loss are characterised by normal or increased numbers of megakaryocytes in the bone marrow. In contrast, the thrombocytopenias reflecting decreased production are associated with reduced marrow megakaryocytes (except in the megaloblastic anaemias where thrombopoiesis is ineffective).

Idiopathic thrombocytopenic purpura (ITP)

The diagnosis of ITP depends both on the demonstration of an isolated thrombocytopenia with increased numbers of megakaryocytes in the bone marrow and on the exclusion of known causes of secondary autoimmune thrombocytopenia (Table 4.1).

Acute and chronic forms of the disease occur. The acute form is the usual type in children and frequently has a self-limited course, spontaneous remission often occurring in days to weeks. In contrast, chronic ITP has an insidious onset and may persist for months to years.

Both forms of the disease are characterised by thrombocytopenic bleeding (skin petechiae, purpura and bruising, and mucosal bleeding). Splenomegaly and lymphadenopathy are not features of the diseases.

If symptomatic, the thrombocytopenia is treated with high-dose steroids. If a good response is achieved, the dose of steroid is rapidly reduced and stopped. In acute ITP, withdrawal of steroid is often followed by sustained remission, but in the chronic form symptomatic thrombocytopenia usually recurs. Splenectomy is indicated if marked thrombocytopenic bleeding persists despite an adequate trial of steroid, or if repeated withdrawal of steroid is followed by recurrence of symptomatic disease. Most patients will respond to splenectomy, but in those in whom

Table 4.1

Causes of Thrombocytopenia

Decreased production
    Selective megakaryocyte depression due to drugs (e.g. gold, etc.)
    General marrow aplasia or hypoplasia
    Marrow infiltrations
    Megaloblastic anaemias
    Alcohol

Increased destruction
    Primary autoimmune (acute or chronic ITP)
    Secondary autoimmune (e.g. infectious mononucleosis, lymphoproliferative disorders, SLE)
    Alloimmune (e.g. neonatal thrombocytopenia, Chapter 3)
    Drug-induced immune (e.g. quinine in tonic water, sulphonamides, etc.)
    Disseminated intravascular coagulation

Abnormal distribution
    Splenomegaly

Dilutional loss
    Massive transfusion

thrombocytopenic problems persist, long-term low-dose steroid and immunosuppressive agents (e.g. azathioprine) should be given.

Qualitative defects in platelets

A variety of defects of platelet function, both congenital and acquired, are known.

Hereditary defects of platelet function

All these defects are rare, but they have been important in pin-pointing the pathways of platelet–collagen and platelet–endothelium interaction. Details of these are beyond the scope of this chapter. The important abnormalities involve failure of:

    adhesion to collagen (Ehlers syndrome)
    adhesion to subendothelium (Bernard–Soulier syndrome, von Willebrand's disease)
    the release reaction (storage pool deficiency)
    aggregation (Glanzman's thrombasthenia).

In von Willebrand's disease there is defective adhesion of platelets to subendothelium. This abnormality is the result of a defect in that part of the factor VIII molecule (VIIIR:WF) necessary for normal platelet adhesion (and for ristocetin aggregation; p. 63). In addition, the coagulant function of factor VIII is abnormal (p. 63).

Acquired defects of platelet function

Such defects are often multiple and may affect both vascular and clotting function. The commonest acquired platelet defect is a result of the effects of drugs; in addition, renal failure, the myeloproliferative disorders, and high levels of FDPs may affect platelet function. Many drugs interfere with platelet function. Important examples include commonly-used drugs such as aspirin, dipyridamole, the penicillins, phenothiazines, tricyclic antidepressants and many nonsteroidal anti-inflammatory compounds. Such drug effects may either themselves result in a bleeding effect (usually mild) or aggravate an existing bleeding tendency. A drug history is therefore essential in the investigation of any bleeding disorder and whenever platelet function studies are being performed. Moreover, some of these drugs may have potential value in the prevention of thrombosis (see Chapter 5).

Disorders of Blood Coagulation

Liver disease and vitamin K deficiency

The most common acquired defect of coagulation is that due to liver disease. The vitamin K-dependent factors (II, VII, IX and X) are synthesised in the liver; deficiencies may develop either from hepatocellular failure or from vitamin K deficiency of whatever cause. In the former case, vitamin K will not correct the haemostatic defect; infusion of the appropriate clotting factor, usually in the form of fresh frozen plasma, is necessary. However, where some hepatocellular function is preserved, but where obstructive jaundice has led to malabsorption of vitamin K, parenteral administration of the vitamin can be expected to produce a beneficial response. In severe liver disease, as well as failure of vitamin K-dependent factors, factor V and fibrinogen levels may also be reduced. Furthermore, the haemostatic defect may be compounded by the development of thrombocytopenia and qualitative abnormalities in platelets. In some patients, disseminated intravascular coagulation and pathological fibrinolysis may further complicate the picture. This leads to consumption of a variety of clotting factors and the appearance of high levels of FDPs in the plasma.

Vitamin K is a fat-soluble vitamin obtained from green vegetables and bacterial synthesis in the gut; its absorption requires the presence of bile salts. The vitamin K deficiency that occurs in obstructive jaundice (as a result of the absence of bile salts from the gut) has already been mentioned, but deficiency may also be due to inadequate dietary intake, malabsorption, or sterilisation of the colon with broad-spectrum antibiotics. Newborn infants are commonly deficient in this vitamin owing to a combination of intestinal sterility and inadequate maternal stores. All these different types of vitamin K deficiency respond to administration of the vitamin, except for the deficiency in premature infants, where liver-cell function is immature and where infusion of fresh frozen plasma may be necessary.

Haemophilia and Christmas disease – haemophilia A (classic) and haemophilia B

These two disorders are indistinguishable clinically and both are inherited as X-linked recessive characteristics.

The incidence of haemophilia is of the order of 1 in 10 000, while Christmas disease is approximately five times less common.

In both diseases, there is a spectrum of clinical severity approximately correlating with the assayed level of coagulation factor in the plasma. The abnormality of blood coagulation manifests itself early in life, probably when the child starts to move about in his cot, and spontaneous and traumatic bleeds continue throughout his life. Despite modern management, there is still a significant mortality rate. The main sites of bleeding are into the joints and muscles, subcutaneous bruising, and haemorrhage after dental extraction and surgery. Less common sites of bleeding include the gastrointestinal and urinary tracts, larynx, tongue and retroperitoneal space. The commonest cause of death is intracerebral bleeding, which may occur spontaneously or after trauma.

In all these different kinds of bleeding, the haemostatic defect can be corrected with an infusion of the appropriate plasma concentrate, which must be continued until complete healing has occurred. In haemophilia, mild to moderate haemorrhage is usually treated by daily infusions of cryoprecipitate (Table 3.5), while severe bleeding or surgery should be covered with twice-daily doses of factor VIII concentrate (Table 3.5) designed to keep the level of factor VIII between 50–100% of the normal value. Haemorrhage in Christmas disease is treated with factor IX concentrates which, because of their longer half-life, can be given less frequently than factor VIII.

In a small number of cases of haemophilia (3–6%), inhibitors to coagulation factors develop, concentrate infusion fails to produce any (or only a transient) rise in factor VIII, and haemostasis cannot be secured. A variety of activated clotting factor concentrates are under trial to attempt to bypass the inhibitor activity.

Complications of therapy for both haemophilia and Christmas disease include hepatitis and a variety of allergic reactions as well as acquired immune deficiency syndrome.

von Willebrand's disease

This hereditary bleeding disorder affects males and females equally and is inherited in an autosomal dominant manner.

In the usual form of the disease (classical von

Willebrand's disease), factors VIIIR:Ag and VIIIR:WF are deficient and, although factor VIIIc is still formed, it cannot function properly in the absence of the other factors (that factor VIIIc is being formed is demonstrated by the fact that infusion of normal or haemophilic plasma produces a sustained rise in factor VIIIc).

In most patients, a capillary-type bleeding defect (attributable to deficiencies of VIIIR:Ag and VIIIR:WF) predominates, particularly involving the mucous membranes of the gastrointestinal tract and the uterus. In those severely affected, bleeding into joints or muscles may occur.

The diagnosis is established by obtaining an appropriate history and by demonstrating a prolonged bleeding time, defective ristocetin-induced platelet aggregation in the presence of normal aggregation to other agents, and reduced factor VIIIR:Ag and VIIIc activities. A delayed but marked and sustained increase in factor VIIIc activity after infusion of cryoprecipitate confirms the diagnosis and forms the basis of treatment.

Variants of von Willebrand's disease occur, in which factor VIIIR:Ag is present but electrophoretically abnormal.

Use of fibrinolytic inhibitors in coagulation disorders

It is probable that a balance exists between fibrinolysis and blood coagulation and that, in certain circumstances, this may be upset. Inhibitors of fibrinolysis may be useful in reducing bleeding from sites where local fibrinolysis is active (e.g. in the uterus, or after dental extraction, or prostatectomy). The two drugs used are aminocaproic acid and tranexamic acid. There is convincing evidence of their value, but there is also a small risk of the formation of fibrin which may be unlysable as it will incorporate the inhibitor. This has occasionally produced permanent obstruction in the renal tract and, on occasion, obstructive nephropathy; the drugs should not therefore be used for bleeding from the upper genito-urinary tract. There is no evidence of an increased incidence of thrombotic vascular occlusion, although this remains a theoretical possibility.

Defibrination syndrome

The defibrination syndrome is a relatively common cause of bleeding in patients with a variety of illnesses. In defibrination states there is activation of the fibrinolytic system. Increased quantities of circulating plasmin digest circulating fibrinogen as well as fibrin haemostatic plugs. As a result, increased quantities of fibrinogen or fibrin degradation products (FDPs) are present in plasma. Bleeding occurs as a result of the combination of lysis of fibrin haemostatic plugs, low plasma fibrinogen level, and interference with fibrin formation produced by excess FDPs (Fig. 4.5). The combination of low fibrinogen level and increased FDPs gives a useful screening test for diagnosing the defibrination syndrome.

Diseases which may be complicated by the defibrination syndrome are listed in Table 4.2. Activation of the fibrinolytic system may be primary or secondary (Fig. 4.5). *Primary excessive fibrinolysis* is uncommon, but may occur after heart bypass surgery or as a complication of certain carcinomas (e.g. prostate or pancreas). Excess primary fibrinolysis is also produced by therapeutic intravenous infusions of fibrinolytic activators (streptokinase or urokinase), given for treatment of major thrombosis, and their use is frequently complicated by bleeding (see Chapter 5).

Excessive fibrinolysis is much more commonly a *secondary* condition, occurring as a response to disseminated intravascular coagulation (DIC). Many of the conditions listed in Table 4.2 result in widespread activation of the coagulation system. For example, massive tissue injury from major trauma can cause release of large amounts of thromboplastin. Transfusion of incompatible blood may result in acute haemolysis and release of thromboplastins from damaged red cells; in septicaemia, bacterial endotoxin damages leucocytes, again causing release of thromboplastins into the circulation. As a result of widespread thrombin production, there is diffuse formation of fibrin strands and thrombi in small blood vessels. Such widespread fibrin formation causes depletion of platelets, fibrinogen and other clotting factors such as factor V and factor VIII. In addition, there is secondary activation of the fibrinolytic system as a response to the widespread fibrin formation. Bleeding results from the combined effects of activated fibrinolysis, low plasma levels of fibrinogen and other clotting factors, increased FDPs, and thrombocytopenia. Paradoxically, therefore, diseases which cause DIC produce thrombosis initially, but subsequently cause bleeding due to consumption of clotting factors and activation of fibrinolysis.

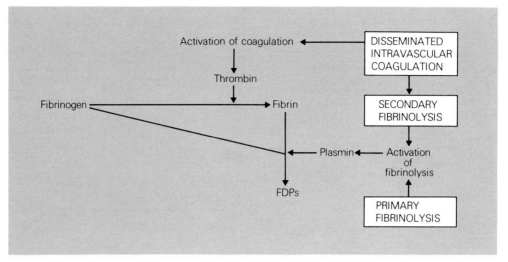

Fig. 4.5 *The defibrination syndrome.*

While bleeding is usually the most obvious clinical feature of DIC, other symptoms are commonly present. Widespread microthrombosis causes tissue ischaemia and organ dysfunction, leading to confusion and coma from brain involvement, hypoxia from lung involvement, and renal failure from kidney involvement. Fibrin strands in capillaries can slice up red cells, resulting in one type of intravascular haemolytic anaemia. Because the red-cell damage occurs in small blood vessels, this is called micro-angiopathic haemolytic anaemia. Red-cell fragments (schistocytes) can be seen on a blood film, and this may lead to the first suspicion of the diagnosis.

In summary, defibrination syndrome should be considered in any sick patient with bleeding, particularly in the clinical situations listed in Table 4.2. Laboratory investigations usually show prolongation in clotting-time tests, particularly the thrombin time; a low platelet count and red-cell fragments on the blood film support the diagnosis. Further laboratory tests may be performed to show excessive fibrinolysis or raised plasma levels of FDPs.

Treatment of defibrination involves: general management; treatment of the disease which caused the coagulation disorder, which is of paramount importance; replacement of clotting factors and platelets; and consideration of antithrombotic treatment. General management consists of treatment of the hypoxia, shock and renal failure which are commonly present in these sick patients, using oxygen, intra-venous fluids, and blood transfusion. Treatment of the disease involves antibiotic therapy in septicaemia, and evacuation of the uterus in placental abruption or the dead fetus syndrome. Replacement of clotting factors and platelets is guided by the results of laboratory tests: whole blood, fresh frozen plasma, cryoprecipitate (which is rich in fibrinogen as well as factor VIII), and platelet concentrates may be indicated. Antithrombotic treatment can be considered if the above measures are ineffective. Heparin (see Chapter 5) is sometimes used, but must be given under careful control since it

---

Table 4.2

Some Conditions Associated with the Defibrination Syndrome

Shock
Septicaemia
Acute haemolysis (including falciparum malaria)
Major trauma
Malignant disease
Major surgery (e.g. cardiac bypass)
Major burns
Antepartum haemorrhage (placental abruption)
Amniotic fluid embolism
Septic abortion
Retained dead fetus
Snake bite

---

may aggravate bleeding. Infusions of antithrombin III can also be considered.

INVESTIGATION

Investigation of the Bleeding Patient

For all patients, it is essential to obtain an adequate history, to perform a physical examination, and to apply a variety of screening tests of vessel, platelet and coagulation function. If any of these screening tests are abnormal, then specific assays are required (Fig. 4.6).

The most important clues are often obtained from a careful clinical history, which should be directed towards answering the following questions. Is the bleeding defect lifelong or of recent onset? Is it a generalised defect or due to a local cause? Is the type of defect suggestive of a vascular, platelet or coagulation defect? Is there a family history, and what is its mode of inheritance?

Patients with a genetic haemostatic abnormality usually present in childhood and often have a preceding family history of bleeding to excess. The origins of bleeding which must be inquired into are: the umbilical cord, circumcision, shedding of milk teeth, tonsillectomy and other childhood operations such as hernia repair, orchidopexy and orthopaedic procedures. The exception to this is the patient with a mild defect who may have been aware of slight excess bleeding in early life, usually after dental extraction, but who receives a major challenge only in later life (e.g. laparotomy or prostatectomy).

In patients with an acquired haemostatic defect, the drug history may prove vital, and the general medical history may reveal important causes of defective

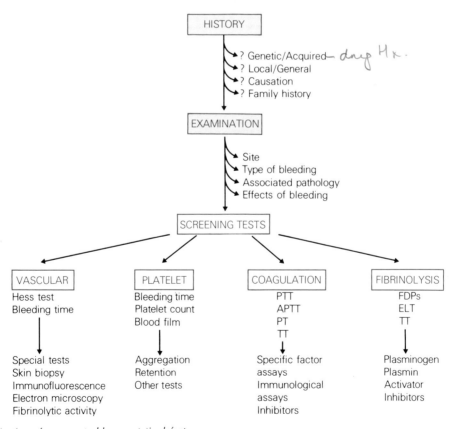

Fig. 4.6 *Investigation of a suspected haemostatic defect.*

haemostasis, such as liver disease, renal failure or malabsorption. The majority of patients sent for routine screening of supposed haemostatic defects have local bleeding as the only feature, e.g. after dental extraction, or excessive menstruation. Even if no other history is available, a panel of screening tests should be done.

General examination of the patient involves definition of the site and type of bleeding, plus a search for signs of associated pathology such as liver disease, renal failure, malignancy, leukaemia, malabsorption, hypersplenism or immune disorders. Evidence should be sought of the effects of previous bleeding into joints, muscles or nerve entrapments. General examination, however, is often remarkably unhelpful and screening tests are also required.

Laboratory Investigation

Tests of haemostasis may be divided into two groups – screening tests, and specific tests which pinpoint the defect (Fig. 4.6). Screening tests are essential because of the large number of patients requiring investigation, and are directed at each of the components of haemostasis, i.e. platelet function (count, bleeding time), vascular function (Hess test and bleeding time, coagulation (activated partial thromboplastin time, prothrombin time and thrombin time), fibrinolysis (fibrinogen level, FDPs and euglobulin lysis time).

Platelet count

Measurement of the platelet count is one of the most valuable laboratory tests, because thrombocytopenia is one of the commonest haemostatic defects seen in clinical practice. When the count is abnormal, examination of platelet morphology on a stained blood film is essential; it may reveal abnormal forms of platelets and also indicate a prime pathology, such as leukaemia. A range from 150–400 × 10⁹/l is normal.

Bleeding time

This test measures the time taken for cessation of bleeding when a cut is made in the skin. It is therefore a measure of platelet adhesion of collagen, platelet-granule release and aggregation, and vessel-wall contraction.

It is prolonged in patients with thrombocytopenia, qualitative platelet defects, and some abnormalities of vascular function.

Various methods of determining the bleeding time have been used in the past, but most laboratories now use one of a range of commercial gadgets which standardise the depth of the cut and are disposable, sterile, and painless. The normal bleeding time is less than 10 minutes.

Hess test

The test consists of applying pressure with a sphygmomanometer cuff to the upper arm (approximately 80 mm Hg for 5 minutes). This increases the pressure in the capillaries and also induces anoxia. In a positive test, a series of purpuric spots appear below the point of application of the cuff. The test is a very crude measure of vascular and platelet function, and is unsatisfactory since it may be positive in normal individuals.

Activated and non-activated partial thromboplastin time (APTT:PTT)

Plasma for all the standard tests of blood coagulation is prepared by adding nine volumes of blood to one volume of sodium citrate, which binds calcium ions and thus acts as an anticoagulant. The partial thromboplastin time (PTT) measures the normality of the intrinsic pathway of blood coagulation (Fig. 4.7). Phospholipid is

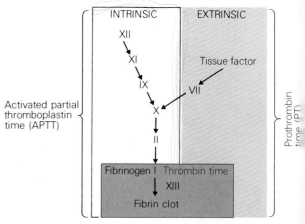

Fig. 4.7 *The parts of the coagulation cascade tested by the prothrombin, activated partial thromboplastin, and thrombin tests.*

added as a source of platelet factor III, and the mixture of plasma and lipid is recalcified. Because of variability in contact activation, it is usual to add a small amount of kaolin suspension to ensure that maximum activation of factor XII to XIIa has occurred (APTT). The normal APTT is 30–40 seconds; it is prolonged in patients with deficiencies of clotting factors XII, XI, IX, VIII, X, V, prothrombin and fibrinogen, and also in patients with circulating anticoagulants. It is normal in patients with factor VII deficiency. If, in the test sample, there are normal prothrombin and thrombin times, factor VIII or IX deficiency is the most likely diagnosis and specific assays of these factors must be done. Failure of kaolin to shorten a prolonged PTT would indicate the presence of an abnormality in the contact mechanism. The presence of an inhibitor is detected by failure of normal plasma to correct the test abnormality.

These tests are relatively simple and sensitive screening tests of the intrinsic system.

Prothrombin time (PT)

This test bypasses that part of the intrinsic coagulation cascade above factor X, and the clotting of the plasma sample is dependent on the concentration of factors VII, X, V, prothrombin and fibrinogen (Fig. 4.7). Equal volumes of test plasma and brain extract are recalcified, and the clotting time is recorded. The normal range obtained varies from laboratory to laboratory; depending on the reagents used, it is between 10–15 seconds. Prolongation of the test-sample clotting time to more than two seconds beyond the control suggests a defect of one of the above factors, provided that no heparin has been given to the patient. A prolonged PT in combination with a normal thrombin time (see below) suggests a deficiency of factors X, V, or prothrombin (APTT also prolonged) or of factor VII (APTT normal), and specific assays of these factors are then indicated.

Thrombin time (TT)

Thrombin is added to plasma in a concentration adjusted to clot normal plasma in up to 15 seconds (Fig. 4.7). Abnormal samples exceed the control clotting time by three seconds or more. The thrombin time is prolonged in patients with fibrinogen defects, whether quantitative or qualitative (dysfibrinogenaemia), but is also prolonged when the thrombin–fibrinogen reaction is inhibited by heparin, paraproteins, or high levels of FDPs.

Fibrinogen/fibrin degradation products (FDPs)

These can be measured by a variety of techniques, most of which have an immunological basis. Normal serum contains < 10 μg/ml fibrin degradation products. Slightly raised values are found in a number of clinical situations (e.g. liver or thromboembolic disease); greatly elevated levels indicate an active fibrinolytic process, such as that seen during therapeutic use of fibrinolytic activators or in cases of fulminant DIC.

Euglobulin lysis time

Dilution and acidification of plasma precipitates euglobulins, which include fibrinogen as well as plasminogen and its activators. The inhibitors of fibrinolysis are removed in the supernatant. The precipitate is redissolved in buffer and clotted with thrombin. The time taken for dissolution (lysis) of this fibrin clot reflects the levels of fibrinogen, plasminogen and activator present.

Fibrinogen

This can be measured in terms of its biological function as thrombin-clottable protein, or by more specific methods. In the former type of assay, spuriously low levels will be found in the presence of thrombin inhibitors (e.g. heparin or FDPs).

Special tests of haemostasis

These are performed in specialised laboratories. Some of the appropriate types of investigation are given in Fig. 4.6. Most of the haemostatic factors can now be assayed directly for activity, using a wide variety of techniques, including radioimmunoassay, and biological function in deficient substrates. Normal variants can also be detected by the use of specific antibodies.

5

Thrombosis

INTRODUCTION

Thrombosis is the formation of a solid mass (thrombus) from the constituents of the blood within the heart or blood vessels during life. Some thrombi give rise to no symptoms, but others produce disability or death by growing sufficiently to block a large blood vessel (e.g. the major artery or vein in a limb) or a smaller but critical blood vessel, such as a coronary artery or cerebral artery. Fragments of thrombi may also break off and block blood vessels downstream (embolism).

Thrombosis concerns the haematologist, who may discover an abnormality in the constituents of the blood in some patients, or may control treatment of thrombosis by drugs which interfere with blood consti-tuents (e.g. anticoagulant drugs). But thrombosis is also of major importance to all doctors, and indeed to society, for thrombosis is now the major threat to life and limb in adults over forty years old. In peacetime, nearly half of British adults will die from one of the three common types of thrombosis:

a. Coronary artery thrombosis, causing myocardial infarction, a common type of heart attack.
b. Cerebral artery thrombosis, causing cerebral in-farction, the commonest type of stroke.
c. Pulmonary thromboembolism; the sudden dis-lodgement of a thrombus which has formed in a large lower limb vein (usually the femoral vein or iliac vein) and its subsequent journey through the right side of the heart to block a large part of the pulmonary arterial tree, and thus obstruct the whole circulation.

Many more patients will suffer non-fatal attacks of thrombosis at these three common sites, or at other less common sites, and some of these attacks will leave them disabled – paralysed, dumb, blind, breathless or limping with a painful, swollen or ulcerated leg. In summary, the well-being and survival of British adults are constantly threatened by thrombosis during the second half of their lifespan. This fact alone should arouse interest in the questions considered in this chapter:

1. What are thrombi made of?
2. Where and why do thrombi occur?
3. How can we treat and prevent thrombosis?

This chapter aims to provide an overview of throm-bosis and its relation to the haemostatic mechanisms outlined in the previous chapter. For the details of diagnosis and management of thrombosis at particular sites, the reader is referred to the other volumes in this series.

STRUCTURE OF THROMBI

We have defined a thrombus as a solid mass formed from the components of the blood within the vascular tree during life. Blood will solidify after death, but the pathologist dissecting a body is able to distinguish a thrombus formed before death from a post-mortem blood clot. The latter resembles the clot formed when a blood sample is placed in a test-tube: it is soft and dark red, and microscopic examination shows a random distribution of red cells and fibrin strands, with occa-sional trapped white cells and platelets. On the other hand, a developing thrombus is firmer to the touch and often partly adherent to the vessel wall. It is paler in colour ('white thrombus'), due to a relative deficiency of red cells, the colour varying from grey to pink. Microscopy shows a laminated structure, layers of massed platelets alternating with layers of fibrin strands and neutrophil polymorphonuclear leucocytes. Red cells are also trapped in varying amounts, but it is evident that in the early development of thrombi there has been selective deposition of platelets, fibrin and white cells. The laminated structure suggests that this has occurred in successive episodes. Once a thrombus has totally blocked a blood vessel, stasis of blood occurs on either side, and further thrombus may grow in either direction. This part of the thrombus, growing in conditions of stasis, is relatively richer in red cells than the initial thrombus, and more closely resembles a test-tube clot or post-mortem clot ('red thrombus').

The structure of thrombi in arteries is quite different from the structure of venous thrombi. Arterial thrombi are rich in platelets and poor in red cells (white thrombi), while venous thrombi are richer in red cells (red thrombi). The different flow conditions in arteries and veins may account for these different structures. In arteries, the high blood flow rates flush away red cells from the site of the thrombosis, leaving the adhesive platelets and leucocytes as the major components of thrombi. In veins, the slow flow rates allow red cells to be incorporated in the network of extending fibrin.

After a thrombus has formed, several processes occur which limit its size and may prevent vessel occlusion or restore vessel patency. These are: (a) retraction of the thrombus; (b) fibrinolysis, which is digestion of fibrin strands by the plasma enzyme plasmin and by other proteolytic enzymes released from the neutrophil polymorphs trapped in the thrombus; and (c) tissue repair ('organisation'), caused by invasion of macrophages and fibroblasts from the vessel wall, which digest the thrombus and convert it into a fibrous plaque covered by endothelium. In arteries, the incorporation of thrombi into the arterial wall as plaques is one mechanism by which atherosclerosis advances. In some arteries and veins that have been totally occluded, these processes may fail to restore the patency of the vessel, which in time shrinks to become a fibrous cord.

CAUSES OF THROMBOSIS

The nineteenth-century German pathologist, Virchow, considered that the factors promoting thrombosis fell into three groups. First, changes in the vessel wall; secondly, changes in blood flow; and thirdly, changes in the blood components. These three groups of causative factors are called Virchow's triad.

The vessel wall can be examined by pathologists for structural abnormalities, and more recently the biochemistry of vessel walls has received much attention. Pathologists have shown that arterial thrombi usually occur at sites of arterial damage, most commonly atherosclerotic plaques. Biochemical abnormalities in these plaques may promote thrombosis; deficiency of prostacyclin, for example, may promote platelet adhesion.

The role of blood flow can be investigated by studying the sites at which thrombosis occurs, and also by studying the effects of alteration of blood flow on thrombosis. For example, thrombosis in the femoral vein is common after hip surgery. It has been shown that the femoral vein is occluded during surgical manipulation, and the resulting venous stasis would favour thrombosis at this site.

Changes in blood components have also been examined. There are similarities between the platelet–fibrin haemostatic plug required to stop bleeding, and the platelet–fibrin thrombus which can kill. Just as haematologists have found defects in platelets, clotting factors, and fibrinolysis that cause abnormal bleeding in some patients (Chapter 4), so they have searched for abnormalities which might cause a swing of the haemostatic balance in the opposite direction to cause thrombosis. One such abnormality is deficiency of the coagulation inhibitor, antithrombin III. Certain families with this deficiency have a greatly increased risk of venous thrombosis. The effects on thrombosis of therapeutic alteration of platelet behaviour, clotting factors, or fibrinolysis may also shed light on whether or not these factors participate in thrombosis.

Finally, studies of large populations of patients with arterial or venous thrombosis may reveal associations with certain characteristics, such as age, sex, obesity, or smoking habits. These risk associations emerging from epidemiological studies may give clues to causative factors.

ANTI-THROMBOTIC DRUGS

Aggregates of platelets and strands of fibrin are major components of thrombi. Development of antithrombotic therapy has logically followed three approaches: inhibition of platelet activity; inhibition of clotting activity; and stimulation of fibrinolytic activity.

Anti-Platelet Drugs

Chapter 4 shows how breach of a vessel wall results in platelets sticking to the exposed subendothelial structures of the vessel wall (adhesion). These activated platelets release adenosine diphosphate (ADP) and other compounds from storage granules into the surrounding plasma, and also convert arachidonic acid from membrane phospholipids into thromboxane A_2 (TXA$_2$) via a series of enzymes, including cyclo-oxygenase. The released ADP and TXA$_2$ induce further platelets to stick to each other and form a platelet mass (aggregation). The aim of anti-platelet therapy is to inhibit adhesion or aggregation, and hence limit the platelet component of thrombi. The agents which are currently being evaluated are aspirin (acetylsalicylic acid), dipyridamole, sulphinpyrazone and prostacyclin (Fig. 5.1).

Aspirin

It has been known for centuries that aspirin relieves pain, fever and inflammation. It is now believed that these effects are due to acetylation of the enzyme cyclo-oxygenase, thus preventing formation of prostaglandins and related compounds which are involved in inflammation. Aspirin also causes bleeding in some individuals, especially haemophiliacs. This was realised by Rasputin, who stopped the aspirin given by previous physicians to the haemophiliac son of Czar Alexander for his sore joints. Consequently there was an improvement in the patient's bleeds, and also in Rasputin's reputation. The explanation of the bleeding is inhibition of platelet cyclo-oxygenase, blocking production of TXA$_2$ and hence impairing platelet aggregation (Fig. 5.1). Unfortunately, aspirin in conventional doses (2–3 g/day) also blocks vessel-wall production of prostacyclin (prostaglandin I$_2$, PGI$_2$) which prevents platelet adhesion and aggregation (Fig. 5.1 and see Chapter 4). This effect reduces the antithrombotic effect of aspirin.

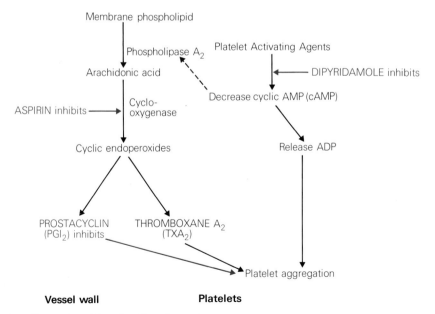

Fig. 5.1 *Anti-platelet effects of aspirin, dipyridamole, and prostacyclin.*

Low-dose aspirin (30 mg/day) selectively blocks platelet formation of TXA$_2$ and aggregation – without inhibiting prostacyclin – but has yet to be evaluated in clinical trials. The main adverse effects of aspirin are epigastric pain, anorexia and nausea; sometimes upper gastrointestinal bleeding can result.

Dipyridamole (Persantin)

Dipyridamole was originally introduced as a vasodilator drug. Its antiplatelet effect (Fig. 5.1) is due to inhibition of the platelet enzyme phosphodiesterase, which results in an increased level of cyclic adenosine monophosphate (cAMP) in platelets, and thus reduces aggregation (Chapter 4). Adverse effects such as headache are due to vasodilatation.

Sulphinpyrazone

Sulphinpyrazone was originally introduced as a treatment for gout because it increases urinary excretion of uric acid. It does not reduce platelet aggregation, but it does reduce platelet adhesion, thus prolonging the life of platelets in the circulation. Like aspirin, it may cause stomach upset.

Prostacyclin (prostaglandin I$_2$, PGI$_2$)

Prostacyclin synthesised by the vessel wall and released into plasma is a vasodilator and also prevents platelet adhesion and aggregation (see Chapter 4). It has recently been synthesised in the laboratory and is currently undergoing trial as an antithrombotic agent. Because of its short half-life, continuous infusion is required. Adverse effects are due to vasodilatation and include headache, nausea, flushing and low blood pressure.

Anticoagulants

The clotting mechanisms of blood may be inhibited by heparin, which must be given by injection since it is not absorbed from the gut; or by oral anticoagulant drugs, of which warfarin is most commonly used.

Heparin

Heparin is a mixture of polysaccharides which contain many sulphate groups and are acidic and negatively-charged. It was discovered in 1916 by McLean, a medical student, in the liver (hepar in Latin), and is now extracted from the lungs and gut of cattle. If heparin is added to a blood sample, clotting is inhibited – 1 unit of heparin keeps 1 ml of blood fluid for 1 hour. Heparin acts as a catalyst: it greatly increases the activity of antithrombin III, the main plasma inhibitor of activated clotting factors (Fig. 5.2).

Low doses of heparin (5000 units twice daily by subcutaneous injection) neutralise activated factor X (Xa), and are effective in prevention of venous thrombosis. Factor X plays a central part in blood coagulation (Fig. 5.2); small amounts of heparin acting here may efficiently prevent excessive thrombin formation by both intrinsic and extrinsic pathways. Low-dose heparin may cause some local bruising, but there is little risk of general bleeding, clotting times are not prolonged, and laboratory monitoring is not required.

Larger doses of heparin (25 000–50 000 units/day) are required for treatment of established thrombosis. Because larger bruises result from subcutaneous or intramuscular injection, these doses are given intravenously, either by intermittent bolus injection (10 000

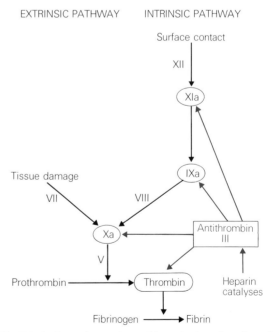

Fig. 5.2 *Anticoagulant actions of heparin. Low-dose heparin neutralises factor Xa. High-dose heparin neutralises thrombin and factors Xa, XIa, and IXa.*

units every 6 hours) or by constant infusion in saline (loading dose 5000 units, then 1000–2000 units/hour). At these doses, heparin neutralises all activated clotting factors (thrombin, Xa, IXa, XIa), prolongs all clotting times, and involves a definite risk of general bleeding. Heparin has a short half-life; intermittent injections cause intermittent effects, and laboratory control is usually not attempted. However, laboratory control of continuous infusions is essential, since patients vary widely in their response to a standard heparin infusion; the activated partial thromboplastin time (see Chapter 4) is commonly used, and the therapeutic aim is an APTT of 1.5–2.5 × normal. If serious bleeding occurs, heparin is stopped and its effect reversed by intravenous protamine sulphate.

Oral anticoagulants

These are coumarin derivatives; the first was dicoumarol, a product of sweet clover fermentation, which caused an epidemic of bleeding amongst cattle in Alberta, Canada in 1921. Warfarin was synthesised at the Wisconsin Alumni Research Foundation (WARF), Madison, USA, and has been used as a rat poison. Oral anticoagulants interfere with synthesis of clotting factors II, VII, IX and X in the liver, at the stage where vitamin K is required; inactive forms of these clotting factors are the result (Fig. 5.3). All stages of the extrinsic pathway are affected, causing prolongation of the plasma prothrombin time (PT). As with heparin, patients vary widely in their response to warfarin, and laboratory control is essential. The therapeutic aim is a PT ratio (patient's time/normal control time) of 2–3. In this range, the coagulation factors are reduced to 5–15% of normal. In the past, different hospital laboratories used different reagents (tissue thromboplastins) when performing the prothrombin time. Because of varying sensitivity of these reagents to the effect of oral anticoagulants, results from different laboratories were not comparable. In Britain, this problem has been solved by issue of a standard reagent (British Comparative Thromboplastin, BCT) to most hospitals, for calibration of local reagents. Results can now be expressed in comparable form. A commercial test with standard reagents (Thrombotest) is used in some hospitals, and the result is expressed as percentage normal activity (therapeutic range 5–15%).

Warfarin is given once daily, starting at a dose of 10

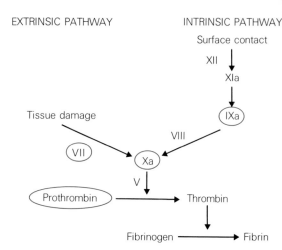

Fig. 5.3 *Anticoagulant actions of warfarin. Warfarin and other oral anticoagulants cause synthesis of inactive forms of prothrombin (factor II) and factors VII, IX, and X.*

mg. It takes 48 hours to act, and the prothrombin time is measured daily from the third day. The dose of warfarin is adjusted to maintain the prothrombin time ratio in the therapeutic range. In different patients, between 2–20 mg daily is required. Once stabilised, tests are performed at less frequent intervals (weeks or months), usually at a special anticoagulant clinic where the tests are done on the spot for a rapid result. Outpatients carry a booklet in which clinic dates, test results, and dose changes are recorded. They are warned to watch for signs of bleeding and to avoid aspirin and alcoholic binges.

It is important that the patient's doctors are aware of the many drug interactions which occur with warfarin; these include antibiotics, anti-inflammatory drugs and anticonvulsants (Table 5.1). Following any changes in medication, frequent laboratory monitoring is required. The patient's dentist should also be notified, since the dose may have to be reduced to avoid bleeding after dental extraction.

Contra-indications to anticoagulants

The anticoagulated patient, like the haemophiliac, is more liable to bleed, and bleeding may occur spontaneously; haematuria and retroperitoneal haemorrhage are two examples. Anticoagulants also cause increased bleeding after trauma, including surgery. While the benefits of anticoagulants in preventing or

Table 5.1

Some of the Many Drugs which Interfere with Warfarin and Other Oral Anticoagulants

Drugs which increase anticoagulant effect	
Broad-spectrum antibiotics	Reduce synthesis of vitamin K by gut bacteria
Liquid paraffin	Reduces vitamin K absorption
Aspirin and other anti-inflammatory drugs, sulphonamides (and sulphonylurea hypoglycaemic drugs)	Displace warfarin from plasma protein binding
Alcohol, chloramphenicol	Inhibit liver enzymes which metabolise warfarin
Drugs which decrease anticoagulant effect	
Barbiturates, griseofulvin	Induce liver enzymes which metabolise warfarin

treating postoperative thrombosis usually outweigh the risk of bleeding, recent surgery or injury to brain, eye or spinal cord contra-indicate anticoagulants because of the risks of intracranial, intraocular or intraspinal bleeding.

Anticoagulants also increase the risk of bleeding from pathological lesions, and are contra-indicated in patients with recent stroke (cerebral infarction as well as cerebral haemorrhage), intracranial or intraspinal tumour, retinal haemorrhages or new-vessel formation (as in diabetic retinopathy), uncontrolled hypertension, aneurysms, acute pericarditis, active peptic ulcer or ulcerative colitis, and ulcerating cancer of the alimentary, urinary or reproductive tracts. Intramuscular injections should be avoided in anticoagulated patients because (as in haemophiliacs) large, painful and crippling haematomas may result.

Patients with haemostatic defects (e.g. thrombocytopenia) are at risk from bleeding, and drugs which inhibit platelet function (aspirin and other anti-inflammatory agents, dipyridamole, sulphinpyrazone) should be avoided, not only for their anti-platelet effect but also because they may cause gastric ulceration.

In pregnancy, warfarin crosses the placenta and may cause a syndrome of fetal malformation as well as fetal haemorrhage. Heparin, which does not affect the fetus, can be used in pregnancy, and patients can be trained to give themselves subcutaneous heparin two or three times a day at home. If subcutaneous heparin cannot be used throughout pregnancy, warfarin can be given between the 16th and 36th week of pregnancy. Heparin is used in early and late pregnancy and is stopped at the onset of labour. After delivery, heparin or warfarin are

restarted, and their use does not contra-indicate breast-feeding.

Treatment of bleeding during warfarin therapy depends on the severity of bleeding. Omitting a dose or reducing the dose may be a sufficient measure for minor bleeding. In severe bleeding the drug is stopped, vitamin K_1 is given intravenously, and clotting factors are replaced by infusion of 2–6 units of fresh frozen plasma.

Fibrinolytic Agents

Anticoagulant drugs reduce fibrin formation: fibrinolytic agents stimulate lysis of fibrin by the enzyme plasmin, and the aim of such therapy is to accelerate removal of the fibrin component of thrombi. Several oral drugs, such as anabolic steroids, increase synthesis of plasminogen activator by venous endothelial cells, and its release into plasma, but there is at present little evidence that these agents are effective in prevention or treatment of thrombosis. On the other hand, there is good evidence that intravenous or intra-arterial infusions of plasminogen activators are able to accelerate lysis of venous and arterial thrombi. The two enzymes which activate plasminogen, and are used in treatment of thrombosis, are streptokinase and urokinase.

Streptokinase and urokinase therapy carry a higher risk of bleeding than anticoagulant drugs. Haemostatic fibrin deposits are lysed as well as fibrin thrombi and, in addition, there is digestion of plasma fibrinogen, resulting in a fall in fibrinogen level and a rise in the circulating FDPs which have anticoagulant effects. Low fibrinogen and high FDP levels bring prolongation of the plasma thrombin time (Chapter 4). This test is monitored during therapy and, if prolonged more than $3 \times$ normal, the infusion rate is reduced. However, laboratory control is less important than careful selection of patients for thrombolytic therapy (p. 76). Serious bleeding should be treated by stopping the infusion and giving a slow intravenous injection of the fibrinolytic inhibitor, tranexamic acid.

SITES OF THROMBOSIS

So far, the structure, causes and treatment of thrombi have been considered in general terms. It must be recognised that thrombi at various sites have dissimilar structures and that the causal factors are probably also different. This is hardly surprising, since veins, arteries, heart chambers and artificial surfaces have very different structures, and the blood elements are exposed to widely varying dynamic forces at these sites. For these reasons, we should not expect that a treatment effective for thrombosis at one site will necessarily be effective elsewhere.

VENOUS THROMBOEMBOLISM

The commonest site for venous thrombosis is in the deep veins of the lower limb, especially the cusp pockets of venous valves and the large venous sinuses within the calf muscles. The initial white thrombus grows until it occludes the vein, resulting in stasis of the whole column of blood and the formation of a long, soft red thrombus. The long red thrombus growing up the femoral vein may detach and travel through the right atrium and ventricle to impact in the pulmonary arterial tree, resulting in pulmonary embolism.

Deep vein thrombosis is uncommon in healthy ambulant people, but common in sick people confined to bed. The risk is greatest in the old, the obese, the patient with a paralysed leg due to stroke or paraplegia, the patient with a splinted leg following fractures or surgery to the hip or knee, patients with heart failure, and patients with widespread cancer. These risk associations suggest that slow blood flow is the major causative factor in deep vein thrombosis. Blood pools in the deep leg veins of these supine and immobile patients, owing to lack of activity of the calf muscle 'pump'. Thrombosis originates where blood flow is slowest – in the valve cusps and venous sinuses.

Examination of the vein wall at the site of leg vein thrombosis reveals no abnormality in the majority of cases. However, venous injury may cause thrombosis in some circumstances (e.g. damage to the femoral or pelvic veins during hip or pelvic surgery respectively). Superficial vein thrombosis and inflammation (thrombophlebitis) may also follow trauma (e.g. at sites of intravenous infusion).

The risk of leg and pelvic venous thrombosis is increased during pregnancy and the puerperium. Possible causes include mechanical factors (compression of pelvic veins by the gravid uterus, enlargement of uterine veins) and the effects of hormones such as oestrogens, which reduce the blood flow and have several effects on the blood (see below).

Two pieces of evidence suggest that activation of blood coagulation also plays a role in venous thrombosis. First, if a segment of vein in an experimental animal is isolated from the rest of the circulation by two ligatures, causing total stasis of blood within the segment, thrombosis does not occur. However, injecting activators of blood coagulation into the segment does result in thrombosis. Secondly, there is good evidence that anticoagulant drugs – heparin or warfarin – are effective in preventing leg vein thrombosis and pulmonary embolism in patients at risk, such as patients undergoing major surgery.

On the other hand, laboratory tests of blood coagulation – clotting times and clotting factor concentrations – are of little help in identifying the patients who will develop thrombosis. Laboratory tests of platelet behaviour or the fibrinolytic capacity of the blood are also of little clinical value. Changes in several of these haemostatic factors occur in groups of patients at risk of venous thrombosis (the old, the sick, cancer patients, postoperative patients, pregnant women and those taking oestrogen-containing contraceptives or other preparations). However, with the single exception of antithrombin III deficiency, no such change has been associated convincingly with thrombosis.

Deficiency of antithrombin III (see Chapter 4), the most important circulating inhibitor of activated coagulation factors, is associated with a greatly increased tendency to venous thrombosis. Antithrombin III deficiency is occasionally found in families as a genetic disorder (thrombophilia), in which inheritance is autosomal dominant. Antithrombin III deficiency is treated with anticoagulant drugs; plasma concentrates of antithrombin III have also recently become available.

Primary polycythaemia is also associated with increased risk of venous thrombosis, and the risk increases as the haematocrit rises (see Chapter 6). Possible mechanisms include increased blood viscosity and increased activation of platelets by the excess red cells.

Prevention of Venous Thromboembolism

Prevention is better than cure, and venous thromboembolism is no exception. Most patients who die of major pulmonary embolism do so without previous symptoms of leg vein thrombosis or of minor pulmonary embolism. In addition, there is little evidence that any treatment of venous thrombosis prevents the chronic symptoms of the post-phlebitic syndrome.

Venous thrombosis may be prevented by mechanical methods or by drugs employed until the patient is ambulant. Mechanical methods aim to prevent stasis in leg veins (e.g. elastic compression stockings). The drug used most widely to prevent venous thrombosis is low-dose heparin (p. 71). Some physicians and surgeons use these prophylactic methods in all patients aged over 40 years who are confined to bed. Others reserve their use for high-risk patients – the old, the obese, patients with varicose veins or a history of venous thrombosis, patients with heart failure or cancer, users of oral contraceptives, and hip surgery patients.

There is little evidence that venous thrombosis is prevented by drugs affecting platelet behaviour (such as aspirin), or by drugs affecting fibrinolysis.

Treatment of Venous Thromboembolism

The clinical diagnosis of venous thromboembolism is unreliable. Only half of patients with a painful or swollen calf have deep vein thrombosis confirmed at venography; in the other half, symptoms are due to a popliteal cyst (Baker's cyst), calf muscle strain or haematoma, or to an unknown cause. Similarly, in many patients in whom pulmonary embolism is suspected because of circulatory collapse, shortness of breath, chest pain, haemoptysis, pleural effusion or lung shadows on chest x-ray, symptoms are due to other pathology in the chest or circulation. Because treatment with anticoagulant drugs carries a major risk of bleeding, it is important to confirm the provisional clinical diagnosis of venous thromboembolism. Venography is the investigation of choice for deep vein thrombosis, and isotope lung scanning is combined with chest x-ray for pulmonary embolism.

Anticoagulants

Although anticoagulants are of value in the prevention of thromboembolic disease in patients at risk, evidence that heparin or warfarin may be beneficial in treatment of established, symptomatic leg vein thrombosis or pulmonary embolism is less convincing. Nevertheless, most clinicians still anticoagulate patients with proven venous thromboembolism unless anticoagulants are contra-indicated. Deep venous thrombosis which extends above the knee carries a particular risk of pulmonary embolism, and most clinicians will give anticoagulants to such patients. Treatment is usually started with intravenous heparin. Oral warfarin may be started at the same time and heparin can then be stopped after 3–5 days, once the prothrombin time indicates adequate anticoagulation by warfarin. Some doctors continue heparin for up to 14 days and delay the warfarin, in the belief that heparin is the more effective antithrombotic agent. However, the risk of bleeding on heparin increases with the duration of treatment, and the short course of heparin is usually effective. It is usual to continue warfarin for at least six weeks to prevent recurrence, and some doctors continue treatment for up to six months. Occasionally, patients develop recurrent venous thromboembolism for no obvious reason; long-term anticoagulation is then given. Some of these patients continue to have recurrent venous thromboembolism despite apparently adequate long-term anticoagulation.

Fibrinolytic agents

Major pulmonary embolism and major (ilio-femoral) deep vein thrombosis appear to be attractive targets for fibrinolytic therapy. Anticoagulants will at best merely prevent further fibrin deposition, whereas fibrinolytic therapy with streptokinase or urokinase has been shown (by repeated venography and angiography) to induce rapid lysis of thrombi and emboli. Paradoxically, however, fibrinolytic therapy has not been shown to be better than anticoagulant therapy in preventing death from pulmonary embolism, or the post-phlebitic syndrome. All the contra-indications to anticoagulant therapy apply, and symptoms should have been present for less than 36 hours (the fibrin in old thrombi is relatively resistant to plasmin digestion). Postoperative patients with venous thromboembolic disease are at particular risk of haemorrhage at the surgical site. In addition, patients over 60 years old are rarely treated because of the risk of intracranial bleeding from aneurysmal or diseased cerebral arteries. Furthermore, the therapy is expensive. For all these reasons, it is rarely employed.

CARDIAC THROMBOEMBOLISM

There are three common sites of origin of cardiac thromboembolism: atrial thrombus in patients with heart failure, especially those with atrial fibrillation or mitral valve disease; thrombosis on artificial heart valves; and ventricular thrombosis overlying an area of myocardial infarction.

Atrial thrombi, like venous thrombi, are usually rich in red cells (red thrombi), and slow blood-flow is again believed to be the main causal factor. They form in the dilated atria of patients with heart failure or mitral valve disease, especially if atrial fibrillation abolishes effective atrial contraction. Long-term anticoagulation with warfarin, which appears to reduce the incidence of thromboembolism in patients with mitral valve disease, should be considered in all such patients. Whether anti-platelet agents are effective is not known.

Thrombi on artificial heart valves are rich in platelets and contain few red cells. Two factors appear to be of importance in thrombus formation. First, artificial surfaces do not have the antithrombotic properties of endothelium (including production of prostacyclin, which inhibits platelet adhesion and aggregation). Secondly, abnormal flow patterns produced by artificial valves result in high shearing forces, which can activate platelets either by direct mechanical effect or by lysis of red cells and release of ADP which aggregates platelets. Although modern materials and designs have reduced the risk, thromboembolism remains a hazard, especially after mitral valve replacement. Long-term anticoagulation with warfarin appears to reduce the risk and is standard practice for artificial mitral valves. The addition of either dipyridamole or aspirin to warfarin has been reported to reduce the risk further.

Ventricular thrombi form on the endocardium covering a myocardial infarct (mural thrombi). Factors favouring thrombosis include the wall damage itself, and possibly also stasis due to flow disturbance from failure of dead muscle to contract. Anticoagulation reduces the incidence of thrombosis, but most clinicians do not use anticoagulants routinely in myocardial infarction (see below). There is no evidence that anti-platelet agents are of benefit.

The most common and distressing result of cardiac thromboembolism is a stroke from cerebral infarction. While anticoagulation is frequently considered for the prevention of further emboli, immediate anticoagulation carries the risk of fatal bleeding into the softened infarcted brain. Anticoagulation should therefore be delayed for some weeks.

ARTERIAL THROMBOEMBOLISM

Arterial occlusion may be due to cardiac thromboembolism or, occasionally, to 'paradoxical' venous thromboembolism (via a patent foramen ovale), but the commonest cause of arterial occlusion is arterial thrombosis. Thrombosis may start at the site of occlusion, or embolise from a proximal artery to a distal artery.

Unlike venous thrombi, arterial thrombi contain relatively few red cells (white thrombus) and almost always occur on abnormal artery walls. Occasionally they occur after arterial wall injury from trauma, arterial catheterisation, or misplaced intravenous injections. However, most arterial thrombi occur spontaneously on atherosclerotic lesions.

Thrombi do not only complicate atherosclerotic lesions; they also contribute to their growth, being incorporated into the arterial wall intima and covered with proliferating endothelium. Platelets have been shown to secrete a growth factor which stimulates proliferation of smooth muscle cells in the arterial wall, and this may be another mechanism by which platelets promote atherosclerosis.

Several changes in platelet behaviour, coagulation factors, and fibrinolysis have been described in patients with arterial thrombosis, but their significance is not known.

Two haematological abnormalities are definitely associated with increased risk of thrombosis. Primary polycythaemia is associated with increased risk of arterial as well as venous thrombosis, and treatment of the high haematocrit reduces the risk (see Chapter 6). Thrombocythaemia (see Chapter 6) is associated with ischaemia of the digits and transient cerebral ischaemia; it is presumed that the high platelet concentration results in spontaneous aggregation in small arteries. Symptoms usually respond to treatment with aspirin, which inhibits platelet aggregation.

Prevention and Treatment of Arterial Thromboembolism

Alteration of risk factors

This includes such measures as advice against smoking and treatment of hypertension.

Anti-platelet drugs

Platelets are prominent in arterial thrombi, and during the past decade several large, long-term trials of aspirin, dipyridamole and sulphinpyrazone in the prevention of arterial thromboembolism have been initiated. The evidence available to date suggests that, in patients with transient cerebral ischaemic attacks, aspirin (1.2 g/day) reduces the frequency of attacks and the risk of progression to completed stroke and death. The results of trials with patients with myocardial infarction have been conflicting, and further studies are required. There is as yet no evidence that anti-platelet drugs are of benefit to patients with a completed stroke or peripheral arterial disease.

Anticoagulant drugs

Fibrin is also a major component of arterial thrombi, but there is less evidence that anticoagulant therapy is of benefit in arterial thrombosis, compared with its use in venous or cardiac thrombosis. Several studies have reported benefit in transient cerebral ischaemic attacks and in myocardial infarction, but the design and the size of these studies have not yet been adequate to convince most clinicians that routine anticoagulation is indicated. Anticoagulants are contra-indicated in a completed stroke because of the risk of intracranial bleeding. Heparin is commonly given to patients with acute occlusion of limb arteries, but benefit is not proven. There is no evidence that anticoagulants are of benefit in chronic angina or peripheral arterial disease.

Fibrinolytic agents

In acute myocardial infarction, streptokinase infusion has been shown to lyse coronary thrombi, and some studies have suggested an improved mortality rate. As with anticoagulants, the design and size of these studies have not convinced clinicians that routine streptokinase therapy is indicated. Acute thromboembolism of peripheral arteries has also been successfully treated with streptokinase, but surgical removal is usually preferred.

Fibrinolytic agents are contra-indicated in stroke because of the risk of intracranial bleeding.

6

The Malignant Haematological Disorders

INTRODUCTION

Many of the haematological disorders discussed elsewhere in this volume are clearly understood and have well-recognised and effective treatments. Such disorders include the deficiency anaemias and haemophilia. The majority of diseases in this chapter, however, are poorly understood and many of them lead to considerable morbidity and mortality.

Malignant transformation may affect any haemopoietic cell-line. The neoplastic changes are usually associated with the accumulation of excessive numbers of cells in the bone marrow or lymphoreticular system. The clinical and pathological manifestations of each type of malignancy depend upon the specific properties of the malignant cells concerned. Sometimes these cells are relatively immature and primitive, e.g. the blasts of acute lymphoblastic leukaemia. On other occasions, the cellular accumulation is of a more mature type, e.g. the small mature lymphocytes of chronic lymphocytic leukaemia. In general, the acute leukaemias and poorly differentiated lymphomas are associated with primitive cells and carry a relatively poor prognosis.

Sometimes the neoplastic cells are mature enough to maintain some of their functional properties. Thus in myeloma the neoplastic plasma cell population usually secretes an immunoglobulin. These antibody molecules are of a single type, as the plasma cell population that secretes them is derived from a single parent plasma cell. The myeloma cells originate from a single *clone* and produce a monoclonal antibody. The loss of cellular heterogeneity, or establishment of monoclonality, is an important marker for many neoplastic haematological diseases.

Confirmation of the clonal nature of leukaemia has come from studies of isoenzymes of G6PD (p. 38) in leukaemic cells. In heterozygous females, who would normally be expected to have a mixture of two isoenzymes in their leucocytes (depending on the random activation of X chromosomes expressing the gene coding for either isoenzyme type), the leukaemic cells have expressed a single enzyme type, suggesting their derivation from a single parent cell.

General Features Shared by Malignant Haematological Diseases

In general, malignant haematological cells proliferate at a slower rate than normal cells, but their proliferation and maturation are not controlled in the normal way. As a result, malignant cells accumulate in bone marrow, spleen and lymph nodes. The resulting impairment of bone marrow function may lead to anaemia, neutropenia, and thrombocytopenia. Certain types of malignant cell have a predilection for particular organs. Thus, in chronic lymphocyte leukaemia (CLL) it is usual to find generalised enlargement of the lymph nodes before severe marrow infiltration occurs. Such enlargement of nodes is unusual in acute myeloid leukaemia (AML). In the T-cell variant of acute lymphoblastic leukaemia (ALL), a mediastinal mass (thymic enlargement) is commonly found.

Cytotoxic Drug Treatment in Haematological Malignancies

The general aim of cytotoxic therapy is to kill malignant cells without producing excessive damage of normal cells.

Concept of pulse chemotherapy

Unfortunately, all cytotoxic agents have some deleterious effects on normal cells. The most important of these effects is marrow depression. Provided that the patient can be supported through a period of marrow suppression caused by chemotherapy, normal haemopoietic cells will usually regenerate faster than malignant cells. Because of this, powerful chemotherapy is usually 'pulsed', with repeated courses of a few days' treatment interspersed with periods of rest to allow marrow recovery.

Concept of combination drug regimens

Different cytotoxic drugs act at different stages of the cell cycle. The division of malignant cells is not synchronised, so the tumour tissue will contain cells at all stages of the cell cycle. Therefore, to maximise cytotoxic effect, it is useful to give several different drugs simultaneously, acting at different stages of the cell cycle. This also allows smaller doses of each individual drug to be used than would be the case in single-agent therapy, so that specific toxic effects are minimised.

Common toxic effects of chemotherapy

Cytotoxic drugs affect all rapidly-dividing tissues, but their effects on the bone marrow and gut are particularly important. Marrow depression results in anaemia, neutropenia and thrombocytopenia, while intestinal toxicity is manifested as vomiting, nausea and diarrhoea. When high-dose parenteral therapy is being given, vomiting may be mediated through central mechanisms, and prophylactic anti-emetics such as metoclopramide or prochlorperazine are administered. Temporary alopecia is a frequent accompaniment of high-dose therapy and it is a kindness to provide a wig, particularly for female patients. A clear explanation of the aims and expected side-effects (Table 6.1) of chemotherapy should be given to patients.

How cytotoxic drugs work

Cytotoxic drugs may be grouped according to their mode of action (Table 6.1).

The alkylating agents, of which mustine was the first example, act by generating highly reactive chemical groupings within the cell (free radicals), which cause cross-linking and breakage of DNA strands. Chlorambucil, cyclophosphamide, busulphan and melphalan are frequently-used examples of this group of drugs.

The antimetabolite group of drugs exert their cytotoxic action by blocking essential metabolic pathways in the cell. Cytosine arabinoside, a synthetic pyrimidine nucleoside, interferes with nucleotide synthesis, resulting in the production of a deformed and inactive DNA helix. Methotrexate specifically inhibits the enzyme dihydrofolate reductase, which is required to convert dihydrofolate to tetrahydrofolate, an essential step in the cell's folate metabolism. Thioguanine and mercaptopurine are purine analogues which block DNA synthesis.

The anthracycline antibiotics, daunorubicin and adriamycin, by incorporation into the DNA helix, inhibit DNA and RNA synthesis and are among the most powerful cytotoxic agents.

Vincristine and vinblastine cause arrest of mitosis in metaphase by poisoning the microtubular spindle apparatus so important in mitosis.

Methods of administration

The usual routes of administration of the commonly used cytotoxic drugs are shown in Table 6.1. Some are inactive when given orally. These must therefore be given parenterally and, in the case of the anthracyclines and vinca alkaloids, intravenously since they cause local tissue necrosis if extravasated. The different routes of parenteral administration do not necessarily result in an identical therapeutic effect. For example, subcutaneous cytosine arabinoside and intrathecal methotrexate have more prolonged systemic effects than identical doses given intravenously.

Table 6.1

Cytotoxic Agents Commonly Used in Malignant Haematological Disorders

Agent	Mechanism of action	Commonly used in	Specific side-effects	Route
Anthracyclines e.g. daunorubicin and the more potent hydroxydaunorubicin or Adriamycin	Antibiotic	Part of combination therapy for AML and lymphomas	Cardiac toxicity Colours urine, saliva, and tears red	i.v.
Bleomycin	Antibiotic	Hodgkin's disease and non-Hodgkin's lymphoma	Pulmonary fibrosis Skin rashes	oral/i.m./i.v.
Chlorambucil	Alkylating agent	Chronic lymphocytic leukaemia	—	oral
Cyclophosphamide	Alkylating agent	Part of combination therapy for CLL, lymphomas, and in high doses for preparation of marrow transplant recipients.	Chemical cystitis at high doses	oral/i.v.
Busulphan	Alkylating agent	Chronic myeloid leukaemia	Pulmonary fibrosis Cytopenic effect persists after cessation of drug	oral
Melphalan	Alkylating agent	Myeloma		oral
Mustine	Alkylating agent	Hodgkin's disease	Vomiting	i.v.
Cytosine arabinoside	Antimetabolite	Part of combination therapy in AML and ALL	—	i.v./s.c./i.t
Thioguanine	Antimetabolite	Part of combination therapy in AML and ALL	—	oral
Mercaptopurine	Antimetabolite	Part of maintenance therapy in ALL and some lymphomas	—	oral
Methotrexate	Antimetabolite	Part of maintenance therapy in ALL and some lymphomas	Soreness of buccal mucosa (mucositis)	oral/i.m./i.t.
Vinca alkaloids (vincristine, vinblastine)	Mitotic spindle poison	Lymphomas, Hodgkin's disease, and ALL	Peripheral neuropathy (especially vincristine)	i.v.
Prednisone	Lymphocytotoxic Vascular protective effect in thrombocytopenia	Most haematological malignancies	Numerous	oral

i.m., intramuscular; i.v., intravenous; i.t., intrathecal; s.c., subcutaneous.

ACUTE LEUKAEMIA

Acute leukaemia is broadly subdivided into acute myeloblastic leukaemia (AML) and acute lymphoblastic leukaemia (ALL).

Although many of the presenting signs and symptoms are the same for both types of disease, it is important to distinguish between them since treatment and prognosis differ.

Differentiation of AML and ALL

In many cases, simple morphological examination of the peripheral blood and bone marrow will allow accurate diagnosis. Thus significant granulocytic maturation (maturing myeloid cells and marked cytoplasmic granulation of blasts) or lymphoid maturation respectively identify AML and ALL.

In many cases of AML, a variable percentage of the host cells contain rod-like cytoplasmic inclusions known as Auer rods. These structures are derived from myeloid granules and are pathognomonic of AML. In difficult cases, the presence of Sudan black or peroxidase staining in blasts makes the diagnosis of AML. In still more difficult cases, immunological markers may help. In particular, the presence of the nuclear enzyme TdT (terminal deoxynucleotidyl transferase) usually identifies a primitive acute leukaemia as lymphoid in type. In addition, the presence of cALL antigen and traditional T- or B-cell markers indicates a diagnosis of ALL (p. 84).

Aetiology

The aetiology of acute leukaemia is still unclear, but radiation and treatment with cytotoxic drugs are known to predispose to the development of acute leukaemia and other malignancies. A few families with a high incidence of acute leukaemia have been reported, and inherited factors may play a minor part in predisposing to the development of leukaemia. Certain congenital chromosomal disorders, particularly Down's syndrome (Trisomy 21; mongolism), are associated with an increased incidence of acute leukaemia. Furthermore, chromosomal abnormalities are detectable in the majority of cases of acute leukaemia, even in patients without previous congenital chromosomal abnormalities.

Viruses are known to cause acute leukaemia in chickens, cats and other animal species, and it is tempting to postulate their involvement in humans.

Several cases have been reported of relapsed leukaemia in transplant recipients where the leukaemic cells carry the sex chromosomes of the marrow donor. This may imply the transmission of a leukaemogenic factor, or alternatively the bone marrow environment in the recipient may in some way induce leukaemic change in the donor's cells.

Incidence

Acute leukaemia is the commonest malignant disease of children, and in adults it ranks approximately twentieth in order of incidence among the common malignancies. The relative incidence of acute leukaemia with age is shown in Fig. 6.1.

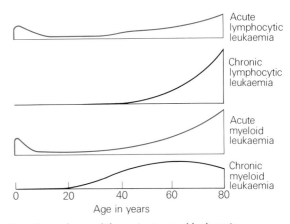

Fig. 6.1 *Incidence of the major types of leukaemia.*

Features Common to the Acute Leukaemias

In both types of acute leukaemia, the bone marrow is filled with primitive blast cells, either lymphoblasts or myeloblasts, which also appear in the peripheral blood in variable numbers. The presence of large numbers of blast cells in the marrow results in impairment of normal haemopoiesis, which in turn results in a combination of anaemia, neutropenia and thrombo-cytopenia.

Lassitude, weakness and shortness of breath are the usual symptoms of anaemia. Pallor may also be noted.

Infections are particularly common in the mouth and around the perineum. Oral thrush is also a common manifestation of neutropenia.

Septicaemias, which commonly originate from the patient's own Gram-negative intestinal flora, are a dangerous complication. Acute bacterial pneumonias are also common, but chest infection may result from organisms rarely associated with infections in immuno-logically-normal individuals. Such infections are known as opportunistic, and are particularly associated with aggravation of neutropenia induced by chemotherapy; typical organisms include *Candida*, *Aspergillus* and *Pneumocystis*. Normally-limited viral infections such as cold sores and shingles may become rapidly genera-lised and associated with severe toxaemia.

Purpura, epistaxis and bleeding from gums and venepuncture sites are the usual signs of thrombocyto-penia. Bone pain and tenderness may also be present.

Treatment

Untreated, acute leukaemia is rapidly fatal; death is due to infection or bleeding, or a combination of the two.

The aim of cytotoxic treatment in acute leukaemia is to induce a remission. Remission induction involves the destruction of large numbers of leukaemic (and normal) cells, and hyperuricaemia may ensue. To prevent this, it is usual to prescribe allopurinol immediately before starting cytotoxic chemotherapy. In remission, the blood and bone marrow return to normal (i.e. normal haemopoiesis is restored), and there is no evidence of leukaemic cells. Without continued cytotoxic treat-ment, relapse will usually occur and, with the aim of preventing this, some form of chemotherapy is con-tinued in remission (maintenance therapy).

Naturally, in a disorder which is commonly fatal, strong psychological support, particularly during the rigours of remission induction, is essential.

ACUTE LYMPHOBLASTIC LEUKAEMIA (ALL)

As can be seen from Fig 6.1, acute lymphoblastic leukaemia is predominantly a disease of childhood, the peak incidence being at 3–5 years of age. In addition to those features common to the acute leukaemias mentioned above, lymphadenopathy and hepato-splenomegaly may be found (Fig. 6.2).

Involvement of the central nervous system in ALL is relatively common. This may present as raised intra-cranial pressure with headache, vomiting and papill-oedema, or with a variety of neurological manifes-tations.

Treatment

With adequate cytotoxic treatment, childhood acute lymphoblastic leukaemia carries a relatively favourable prognosis; about 45% of children survive for 5 years, and it is likely that many of these patients are in fact cured. In adults with ALL, however, the prognosis is much less good.

In ALL, remission can be induced in the majority of patients (90% of children; approximately 70% of adults) with relatively non-toxic drugs such as vincris-tine and prednisone. For remission maintenance, most of the known antileukaemic drugs are given in a cyclical pattern for at least two years at maximum tolerated doses – short of producing dangerous bone-marrow depression.

Sanctuary Disease

In the early cytotoxic schedules for the treatment of ALL, it became clear that many patients, although achieving blood and bone marrow remission, were relapsing with disease in the central nervous system. The blood–brain barrier, so effective in protecting the central nervous system from toxic substances in the circulation, was preventing the passage of cytotoxic drugs. Thus small numbers of residual leukaemic cells persisted in the CNS, causing a later relapse. Cranial irradiation and intrathecal cytotoxic injections have therefore been introduced into more recent schedules of chemotherapy.

The testicles (but not the ovaries) can also act as sanctuaries for leukaemic cells.

ACUTE MYELOBLASTIC LEUKAEMIA (AML)

This is predominantly a disease of adults, though it occurs at all ages (Fig. 6.1). Significant organomegaly is rarer than in ALL, and sanctuary disease is unusual (Fig. 6.2).

Treatment

In AML, remission induction is more difficult than in ALL, and it is usually necessary to produce a substantial period of profound marrow hypoplasia before remission will emerge. During this period the patient is often very unwell and at great risk from infection and/or haemorrhage. Vigorous use of supportive measures such as broad-spectrum antibiotics and blood products – red cells, platelets, granulocytes – is vitally important during this phase of treatment. Although the disease frequently runs a stormy course, reasonable remission rates (70%) are now achieved in AML.

The drugs most commonly used in AML remission induction are thioguanine, cytosine arabinoside and daunorubicin. Maintenance therapy is less successful than in childhood ALL, but probably does serve to prolong the duration of remission. For this purpose, various drug combinations (usually including cytosine arabinoside and 6-thioguanine) have been given, often at monthly intervals.

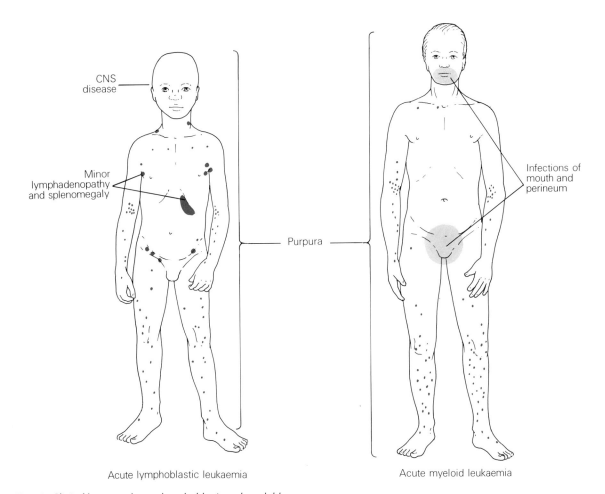

Acute lymphoblastic leukaemia

Acute myeloid leukaemia

Fig. 6.2 *Clinical features of acute lymphoblastic and myeloblastic leukaemia.*

Marrow Transplantation

As AML carries a much worse prognosis than childhood ALL, efforts have been made to find alternative methods of therapy, the most successful of which is marrow transplantation.

Marrow for transplantation is obtained by multiple bone-marrow aspirations from the donor's iliac crest and sternum under a general anaesthetic. The marrow obtained is administered to the recipient by intravenous infusion. The stem cells in the transfused marrow settle in the recipient's marrow cavity and, in a successful graft, will release cells into the peripheral blood in two or three weeks.

Before infusion of donor marrow, the recipient is treated with chemotherapy and total body irradiation; this removes any residual leukaemic cells and produces immunosuppression in order to prevent graft rejection. This causes marrow aplasia and, during the period required for donor marrow regeneration, intensive supportive measures of the type necessary during induction of AML will be needed.

The major problems encountered in marrow transplantation are failure of the transplanted marrow to engraft, rejection of the transplanted marrow, and graft-versus-host disease. Rejection and graft-versus-host disease may be minimised by selecting sibling donors of identical HLA type. The matching of red cell groups and sex are factors less important for obtaining a successful transplant.

The value of performing a marrow transplant in haematological disease must be carefully weighed against the risks involved, bearing in mind the results of conventional chemotherapy. When an HLA-compatible, MLC non-reactive (p. 45) sibling donor is available, it is usual to consider transplantation in AML during first remission, in ALL during second remission, and in aplastic anaemia of severe type (i.e. less than $20 \times 10^9/l$ platelets, less than $0.5 \times 10^9/l$ neutrophils, and when maintenance of an adequate haemoglobin level depends upon transfusion). Transplantation has also been used successfully in the treatment of marble-bone disease and certain rare inherited enzyme disorders. Unfortunately, particularly with the current trend towards small families, only a small minority of patients will have a suitable compatible donor, and this limits the general application of allogeneic transplantation.

Graft-versus-host disease (GVHD) is the result of immunological attack on the recipient's tissues by lymphocytes in donated marrow. This particularly affects the skin, intestine and liver. Usual manifestations are erythematous rash with bullae, diarrhoea and abnormal liver function tests.

The treatment of GVHD depends on suppressing the immunological activity of the donor lymphocytes with steroids, methotrexate, cyclosporin A, or antilymphocyte globulin. Current research is attempting to reduce GVHD by removing donor marrow lymphocytes, through a variety of manipulations *in vitro*, before infusion into the donor.

SUBGROUPS OF ACUTE LEUKAEMIA

Acute myeloblastic and lymphoblastic leukaemias may be further subdivided into immunological and morphological subgroups, some of which exhibit characteristic clinical and pathological features.

Immunological Subgroups of ALL

The lymphoblasts of ALL do not usually express T or B surface markers (p. 15). However, the majority of cases can be positively identified with a specific antiserum – anti-common-ALL (cALL) antiserum. This reagent identifies the common type of childhood ALL (approximately 70% of cases) with a relatively good prognosis. Less common types of ALL that have T or B surface markers (Thy-ALL – approximately 25% cases – and B-ALL – approximately 5% cases) are associated with a poor prognosis. Thy-ALL is often associated with a thymic mass (Fig. 6.3). The blast cells in B-ALL frequently show a characteristic morphological appearance (deep blue cytoplasm with prominent vacuoles), which is also seen in the B cells of Burkitt's tropical lymphoma.

Subgroups of AML

AML is usually subdivided on the basis of morphological appearances rather than immunological surface-marker characteristics.

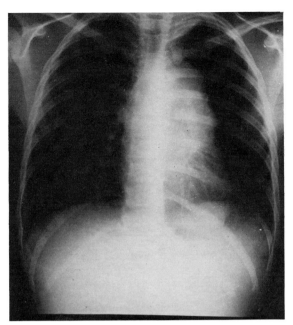

Fig. 6.3 *Mediastinal mass in Thy-ALL. A lateral chest x-ray confirmed the presence of a thymic mass.*

There are six major types:

M1 Undifferentiated AML.
M2 AML with some differentiation into promyelocytes and myelocytes.
M3 Acute promyelocytic leukaemia. Most cells are abnormal promyelocytes rich in procoagulant material, and patients with this variant of AML are particularly liable to develop disseminated intravascular coagulation.
M4 Myelomonocytic leukaemia. There is a mixed proliferation; some of the leukaemic cells are of the neutrophil series, while others possess monocytic characteristics.
M5 Pure monocytic leukaemia, often with skin infiltrates and gum hypertrophy.
M6 Erythroleukaemia. The leukaemic process involves a significant proportion of erythroid precursors.

PRELEUKAEMIA

This is an ill-defined and overlapping group of disorders characterised by increased numbers of myeloblasts in the bone marrow, abnormal myeloid and erythroid maturation, sideroblastic change, and cytopenias of various types. Although progression to acute myeloid (often myelomonocytic) leukaemia is frequent, many cases of preleukaemia remain static for months or even years.

THE CHRONIC LEUKAEMIAS

Like the acute leukaemias, the chronic leukaemias are divided into lymphoid and myeloid types, i.e. chronic myeloid (or granulocytic) leukaemia and chronic lymphocytic leukaemia.

Chronic myeloid leukaemia is usually a disease of middle-aged persons, while chronic lymphatic leukaemia tends to be more prevalent in the elderly (Fig. 6.1). In these chronic leukaemias, relatively mature leucocytes of the lymphoid and myeloid series occur in the blood and bone marrow.

CHRONIC MYELOID LEUKAEMIA (CML)

Anaemia, anorexia and weight loss are the usual presenting symptoms. In contrast to all other types of leukaemia, infection is not a typical presenting manifestation. Splenomegaly is a usual finding, and patients occasionally present with left hypochondrial pain from minor infarctions of an enlarging spleen (Fig. 6.4).

Blood Count

Massive neutrophilia with an increase of immature forms (left shift in the neutrophil series) is the usual blood picture at presentation. The leucocyte count may be high enough to cause a significant increase in blood viscosity, resulting in infarction of vital organs.

Occasionally, a 'leukaemoid-reaction' with gross neutrophilia may be confused with CML. In such cases, an obvious clinical cause for the neutrophilia (e.g. septicaemia) is usually apparent. Doubtful cases may be resolved by means of a neutrophil alkaline phosphatase (NAP) score and chromosome examination. The NAP score is performed by staining a blood film for the

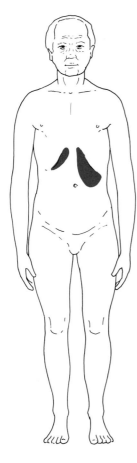

Chronic myeloid leukemia

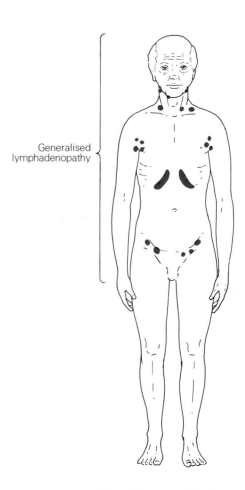

Generalised lymphadenopathy

Chronic lymphocytic leukaemia

Fig. 6.4 *Clinical features of chronic myeloid and lymphocytic leukaemias.*

enzyme alkaline phosphatase and scoring the density of staining in the neutrophils. In CML, the neutrophils are usually deficient in alkaline phosphatase. In leukaemoid reactions, infection, pregnancy, and myeloproliferative disorders other than CML (see below), the NAP score is usually high.

The anaemia is usually normocytic and normochromic, though it may sometimes be slightly macrocytic, especially if a secondary folate deficiency occurs, owing to the massive proliferation of myeloid cells. In addition to the neutrophilia, there are frequently increased numbers of eosinophils and basophils present. The platelet count may be high, normal, or low.

Bone Marrow

This may be difficult to aspirate and is grossly hypercellular with a great increase in numbers of myeloid cells at all stages of differentiation (myeloid hyperplasia).

Philadelphia Chromosome

More than 90% of patients with the clinical and haematological features of CML show a characteristic chromosome abnormality in the cells of the haemopoietic system, namely the Philadelphia chromosome

(Ph[1]) shown in Fig. 6.5. Chromosome 22 has lost part of its long arm, and this portion of chromosome usually re-attaches itself to the long arm of chromosome 9. The Ph[1] chromosome is a useful marker for CML and distinguishes the disease from leukaemoid reactions and other myeloproliferative states; its absence worsens the prognosis in otherwise typical cases.

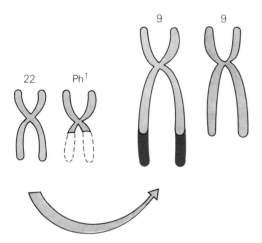

Fig. 6.5 *The Ph[1] chromosome of chronic myeloid leukaemia. The usual 22→9 translocation is shown. The Ph[1] chromosome is the residual small 22nd chromosome.*

Although the NAP score usually returns to normal with effective treatment, the Ph[1] chromosome is always present.

Treatment

Alkylating agents, e.g. busulphan, are the drugs of first choice. Taken orally, their use is associated with a gradual reduction in spleen size and leucocyte count. Unlike other cytotoxic agents, the cytopenic effect of busulphan persists for a few weeks after ingestion is stopped, so that careful monitoring of the patient's haematological state is important; the drug is discontinued when the leucocyte count reaches about $15 \times 10^9/l$.

Accelerated Phase

The chronic phase of CML can usually be controlled by busulphan therapy without difficulty. Eventually, how-ever, all patients enter an accelerated phase of the disease, in which a change in therapy is required. This phase is characterised by worsening anaemia and thrombocytopenia, and increased numbers of blast cells may appear in the blood and marrow. Clinically, bone pains, fever, malaise and weight loss are prominent. Further chromosome abnormalities, in addition to the Ph[1] chromosome, may appear. In some patients, blast cells predominate and the disease resembles acute leukaemia (blast crisis). By means of cytochemi-cal and immunological markers, three varieties of blast crisis have been distinguished: myeloid blast crisis, lymphoid blast crisis, and occasionally mixed myeloid/lymphoid blast crisis.

Identification of the type of blast cells present is important, as lymphoid blast crisis may be treated with relatively non-toxic drug combinations such as vincristine and prednisone. Successful remission induction is rare in myeloid blast crisis of CML.

Less than 25% of patients with CML survive 5 years, though exceptional cases may live for 10 years or more.

CHRONIC LYMPHOCYTIC LEUKAEMIA (CLL)

Patients with CLL frequently present with infections. The increased risk of infection is attributable to a number of factors. First, the disease is usually a neoplastic proliferation of B lymphocytes. B lympho-cytes are responsible for mediating antibody produc-tion and their derangement may result in impairment of humoral immunity, with low immunoglobulin levels. Marrow infiltration, particularly in the later stages of the disease, may also result in neutropenia.

Generalised lymphadenopathy is the commonest clinical finding in patients with CLL. Splenomegaly may also be present, but the degree of enlargement of this organ is much smaller than that seen in CML (Fig. 6.4).

Blood Count

The characteristic finding in the peripheral blood in CLL is a lymphocytosis, the lymphocytes being of normal appearance. Smear cells (lymphocytes ruptured during the making of the film) are commonly seen.

The derangement of B-cell function that has been mentioned as causing immune-paresis may, paradoxically, be manifest as an auto-immune haemolytic anaemia with positive direct antiglobulin test (p. 42) or, more rarely, as immune thrombocytopenic purpura.

Bone Marrow

The mature lymphocytes seen in the peripheral blood are also seen in the bone marrow. In late stages of the disease, this infiltration is severe enough to result in anaemia, neutropenia and thrombocytopenia.

Treatment

Not infrequently, CLL is discovered as an incidental finding in routine blood tests. In such persons a period of clinical observation without cytotoxic treatment is worthwhile, as in many cases progression of the disease is extremely slow. Elderly patients may die of other causes before their leukaemia causes clinical problems.

Chlorambucil is the cytotoxic drug of first choice in CLL. Given orally, it usually results in a satisfactory reduction in the size of lymph nodes, spleen, and lymphocyte count. Occasionally, localised lymphadenopathy (e.g. unsightly enlargement of cervical lymph nodes) may require local radiotherapy.

Advanced stages of CLL, particularly in younger patients, may be successfully treated with combination chemotherapy such as cyclophosphamide, vincristine and prednisone. Prednisone is also an effective treatment for the auto-immune haemolytic anaemia associated with CLL.

Patients who suffer repeated infections may benefit from prophylactic antibiotic therapy, particularly with co-trimoxazole, and from intramuscular injections of polyvalent human gamma-globulin.

THE MYELOPROLIFERATIVE DISORDERS

These disorders are considered together because they consist of a spectrum of diseases with considerable overlap between distinctive clinical entities. One of them, chronic myeloid leukaemia, has already been considered at length above. The others are myelofibrosis, polycythaemia rubra vera, and essential thrombocythaemia.

MYELOFIBROSIS

Myelofibrosis is almost invariably associated with massive splenomegaly. The patient may notice his abdomen enlarging, or the spleen may be felt during routine medical examination (Fig. 6.6). As in CML, infarction of areas of the spleen is common, with resulting left hypochondrial pain, which is often referred to the shoulder if the diaphragmatic peritoneum is involved.

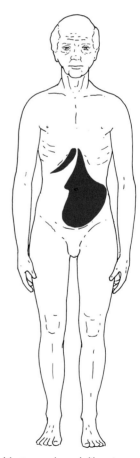

Fig. 6.6 *Clinical features of myelofibrosis.*

Blood Count

Like other causes of marrow infiltration, myelofibrosis may cause a leucoerythroblastic anaemia, i.e. anaemia with myeloid precursors and nucleated red cells in the peripheral blood. The red cells show a characteristic morphological appearance in myelofibrosis – tear-drop or pear-shaped cells (tear-drop poikilocytosis).

Bone Marrow

The pathognomonic finding in myelofibrosis is an increase in marrow reticulin (the scaffolding that supports the cellular elements of the marrow) and, eventually, extensive fibrosis of the marrow cavity. This results in a 'dry tap' when marrow aspiration is attempted, and a trephine marrow biopsy is usually necessary to establish the diagnosis.

Some cases of CML have modestly increased marrow reticulin (rendering them more sensitive to chemotherapy) and some cases of myelofibrosis have high leucocyte counts with left shift. However, the absence of a Ph^1 chromosome and a high LAP score distinguish myelofibrosis from CML.

Extramedullary Haemopoiesis

An important pathological feature of the myeloproliferative diseases, especially myelofibrosis, is the finding of myeloid precursors, erythroblasts and megakaryocytes in the liver and spleen.

Treatment

When therapy is necessary, it is usually of a supportive nature. Folate deficiency often develops as a result of the rapid cellular turnover in the marrow, and it is routine to prescribe oral folic acid supplements. The anaemia may be corrected by the judicious use of blood transfusion.

The massive splenomegaly contributes to the anaemia by sequestering red cells and by increasing the plasma volume (leading to haemodilution). This effect of the spleen may be quantified by ^{51}Cr radiolabelling studies (p. 36). Counting the isotope's activity over the spleen reveals the degree of splenic sequestration of the red cells. Radioactive iron (^{59}Fe) may also be injected in order to provide an estimate of the amounts and sites of red cell precursors, which incorporate the radiolabelled iron into haemoglobin. Although the results of ferrokinetic studies should be interpreted with caution, the demonstration of a major splenic pooling effect, with minor or only moderate splenic extra-medullary haemopoiesis, would encourage splenectomy, provided that the patient is not too old or frail. Each patient must be individually assessed, weighing the advantages of splenectomy against its risks.

The platelet count in myelofibrosis may be low, normal or high. Even when the count is satisfactory, functional abnormalities of platelets may be revealed by platelet aggregation studies.

Chemotherapy has a small part to play in the management of myelofibrosis, but may be of benefit in those patients whose leucocyte count is raised, whose marrow shows relatively little fibrosis, and whose platelet count is not depressed. In such patients, spleen size and marrow fibrosis may be reduced by chemotherapy. Busulphan is the cytotoxic agent generally used.

POLYCYTHAEMIA

True polycythaemia is an increase in the red-cell mass. The red-cell count, haemoglobin, and packed cell volume are usually similarly increased. Pseudopolycythaemia may be seen when dehydration occurs from any cause, such as diarrhoea, vomiting, fever or diuretic therapy.

True polycythaemia may be primary or secondary. Secondary polycythaemia occurs in conditions leading to tissue hypoxia, with compensatory increase in haemoglobin and oxygen-carrying capacity of the blood mediated via appropriately elevated levels of erythropoietin. Such disorders include emphysema, chronic bronchitis, pulmonary fibrosis and congenital cardiovascular anomalies associated with a right-to-left shunt (particularly Fallot's tetralogy). A physiological polycythaemia is present in the newborn and in persons living at high altitudes. The oxygen-carrying capacity of the blood is increased in polycythaemia, but blood viscosity is also increased, and there comes a critical point at which increasing red-cell count produces no further increase in oxygen delivery to the tissues, since the viscous blood flows so slowly. Thus many cases of Fallot's tetralogy benefit from judicious venesection, particularly if the haemoglobin is over 20 g/dl. The correct level of haemoglobin is best found by noting the patient's subjective improvement, since there is no clinically acceptable or practical method of quantifying tissue oxygen delivery.

Secondary polycythaemia may also result from inappropriate production of erythropoietin-like material by a variety of tumours, including renal carcinoma, malignant hepatoma, cerebellar haemangioblastoma and uterine fibroids. Secondary polycythaemia may also be associated with certain non-neoplastic renal disorders such as simple cysts and polycystic kidney.

When none of the causes of secondary polycythaemia is present, and when the increased erythropoiesis represents a primary myeloproliferative disorder, the polycythaemia is of primary type and is known as polycythaemia rubra vera. Here the marrow is no longer under the control of erythropoietin, and erythropoietin levels are low.

Clinical Features

In polycythaemia rubra vera, the usual presenting symptoms are headache, dizziness and vertigo. Not infrequently, a vascular thrombosis is the initial manifestation of the disorder.

A dusky red complexion is usual, and itching of the skin is a frequently associated complaint, particularly on exposure to hot water. A minor degree of splenomegaly is a frequent finding (Fig. 6.7). Hypertension is also often noted.

There is a high incidence of peptic ulcer in patients with polycythaemia rubra vera, and the erythroid hyperplasia leads to a predisposition to gout.

Blood Count

Polycythaemia is associated with an increased haemoglobin, packed-cell volume and red-cell count. In polycythaemia rubra vera, a neutrophil leucocytosis and an increased platelet count are also commonly found; these are often a useful clue in distinguishing primary from secondary polycythaemia. In addition,

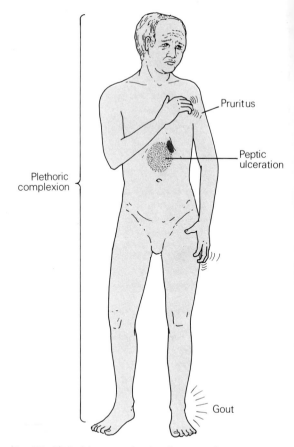

Pruritus

Peptic ulceration

Plethoric complexion

Gout

Fig. 6.7   *Clinical features of polycythaemia rubra vera.*

the ESR is commonly less than 1 mm/hr in primary polycythaemia, and the NAP score is raised. Patients with polycythaemia rubra vera are quite frequently iron deficient, and this may sometimes cause the haemoglobin to be within normal limits despite an increased red-cell mass.

In order to distinguish true polycythaemia from pseudopolycythaemia, it is usual to perform red-cell mass and plasma-volume estimations. An aliquot of the patient's red cells are labelled with ^{51}Cr and re-injected into the circulation. After allowing time for mixing and equilibration, a venous sample is taken. If the body's red-cell mass is high, the isotopically labelled red cells will be heavily diluted, resulting in a low radioactivity count in the blood sample. If the red-cell mass is low, then dilution of the labelled cells will be less, with higher radioactivity counts in the venous sample. The plasma volume may be measured by a similar dilutional method using ^{131}I-labelled albumin.

Bone Marrow

Erythroid hyperplasia is found in the marrow. In polycythaemia rubra vera, an increase in numbers of megakaryocytes, as well as myeloid hyperplasia and a modest increase in reticulin, are also frequently present.

Treatment

Venesection is the usual initial treatment. This rapidly restores the haemoglobin to normal levels, but carries the potential disadvantage of aggravating any thrombocythaemia and iron deficiency present.

Thus, methods of inhibiting marrow erythropoiesis are necessary. The usual method is to administer ^{32}P by intravenous injection. The phosphorus enters equilibrium with the bone phosphate pool, thereby irradiating the bone marrow. This treatment has been criticised because of suggestions that the marrow irradiation may predispose to the development of leukaemia. However, the leukaemogenic risk of moderate doses of ^{32}P is probably low and, in many cases, the development of acute leukaemia is a manifestation of the myeloproliferative state rather than of marrow irradiation. Polycythaemia rubra vera may also develop into myelofibrosis. Cytotoxic drugs such as busulphan can be used to inhibit marrow erythropoiesis.

ESSENTIAL THROMBOCYTHAEMIA

The major abnormality in the blood in primary (essential) thrombocythaemia is a grossly elevated platelet count, often over 1000×10^9/l (normal $150–400 \times 10^9$/l).

Primary thrombocythaemia must be distinguished from other causes of thrombocytosis, such as bleeding, infection and carcinoma.

Although increased in number, the platelets in essential thrombocythaemia are often qualitatively abnormal, and occult gastrointestinal bleeding with secondary iron deficiency is common. Paradoxically,

however, patients with essential thrombocythaemia may also suffer thrombotic incidents.

Therapy is directed at reducing the platelet count. The platelets may be physically removed from the blood by thrombopheresis, using a centrifugal cell separator. This is only a temporary solution, however, and most patients receive busulphan or ^{32}P which returns the platelet count to normal levels. Platelet function approaches normality as the count is reduced.

MYELOMA

This disorder is characterised by a malignant proliferation of plasma cells in the medullary cavity. Very rarely, this proliferation may be localised to one site (solitary plasmacytoma). Usually, however, the plasma cells infiltrate all parts of the marrow (multiple myeloma or myelomatosis).

Clinical Features

The clinical effects of this infiltration depend upon the displacement of normal haemopoietic cells, the elaboration of a monoclonal antibody (or paraprotein), and production of an osteoclast-stimulating factor. The marrow infiltration results in anaemia, neutropenia and thrombocytopenia, any of which may produce presenting symptoms.

The physical properties of the paraprotein may produce specific clinical manifestations. For example, IgA paraproteins, because of their tendency to polymerise (p. 11), have a high intrinsic viscosity and may cause the hyperviscosity syndrome. This syndrome is characterised by weakness, dependent oedema, engorgement of retinal vessels, and bleeding from the mucous membranes of nose and mouth. Plasmapheresis may be usefully employed to remove the abnormal protein in such cases.

The elaboration of osteoclast-stimulating factor by the plasma cells results in bone resorption, with bone pain, general or localised rarefaction of bone (Fig. 6.8), pathological fractures, and hypercalcaemia. The hypercalcaemia may cause polydipsia, polyuria, weakness and constipation. Hypercalcaemia, dehydration, tubu-

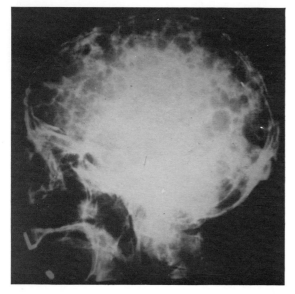

Fig. 6.8 *The skull in a case of multiple myeloma. Numerous lytic lesions can be seen.*

lar precipitation of Bence-Jones protein (see below), hyperuricaemia and deposition of amyloid may lead to renal failure.

Blood Findings

In myelomatosis, a pancytopenia with a leucoerythroblastic blood film is frequently found. The paraprotein causes rouleaux formation, a high ESR, and characteristic blue background staining on the blood film.

Biochemical investigations will show raised globulin; protein electrophoresis will demonstrate a monoclonal peak (Fig. 6.9); and immunoglobulin estimation will reveal the type of paraprotein being secreted and the suppression of the other immunoglobulin classes.

In myeloma, the monoclonal protein is of a particular immunoglobulin class and of a single light-chain type (p. 11). The frequency of occurrence of different classes of paraprotein reflects the relative amounts of the different types of immunoglobulin found in the serum. Thus IgG myeloma is the commonest type of myeloma, IgA disease is less frequent, and IgD and IgE myelomas are rare. IgM paraproteinaemia is usually associated with lymphoid (e.g. Waldenström's macroglobulinaemia) rather than plasmacytoid proliferations.

Free light chains (of a single light-chain type) may be produced in all types of myeloma; being small, the molecules do not accumulate in the serum and are excreted in the urine. This Bence-Jones protein (named after its discoverer) has the unusual property of precipitating when the urine is heated, only to dissolve again when the urine is boiled, but in modern practice it is usually detected by electrophoresis of concentrated urine. In some myeloma cases, Bence-Jones protein is the only one produced; these are called Bence-Jones myelomas.

A paraprotein may sometimes be found in the sera of elderly persons without underlying myeloma (benign monoclonal gammopathy). This is generally of low concentration (< 10 g/l), is not associated with depression of other immunoglobulins, and remains at constant level over several years of observation.

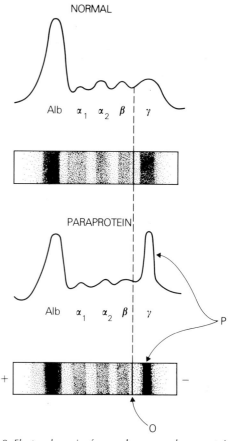

Fig. 6.9 *Electrophoresis of normal serum and paraprotein-containing serum. O = origin or point of application of serum; P = paraprotein.*

Bone Marrow

Increased numbers of plasma cells (normally less than 5%) are observed, and these frequently show abnormal morphological features such as multinuclearity.

Treatment

Melphalan is the most frequently used agent in myeloma; it is generally given orally in intermittent courses, and is usefully combined with prednisone when hypercalcaemia, bone pain, or thrombocytopenia are present. Caution must be exercised in the dosage of melphalan when renal failure is present. Hypercalcaemia is treated by vigorous rehydration and steroids. The cytotoxic agent mithramycin, given by intravenous infusion, inhibits osteoclast activation and may be useful in patients with severe bone pain or refractory hypercalcaemia. In the low doses used to obtain this effect, there is little cytotoxic action on the myeloma cells.

Myelomatosis is invariably fatal, the median survival being $2\frac{1}{2}$ years.

HODGKIN'S DISEASE

Although the aetiology of this disease is still uncertain, great advances have recently been made in its treatment. It commonly afflicts young and middle-aged adults, being commoner in men. As with many other neoplastic haematological diseases, occasional reports of time–space clustering have been made. There is, however, no definitive proof as yet of a viral or other infectious cause for Hodgkin's disease.

Clinical Features

The disease usually arises in a single lymph gland group and then spreads to adjacent lymph nodes, spleen, liver, and bone marrow. Often it is the cervical lymph nodes that are first affected, a lump in the neck being the initial presenting symptom. Pruritus and, rarely, alcohol-induced pain in affected nodes are characteristic but unexplained phenomena. With advancing disease, systemic symptoms make their appearance, particularly weight-loss, sweating, anorexia and fever. Sometimes pyrexia persists for a few days and then disappears, only to return a few weeks later (Pel-Ebstein fever).

Blood Count

A normocytic, normochromic anaemia with raised ESR is the commonest haematological abnormality in Hodgkin's disease. Occasionally, in addition to this 'anaemia of chronic disease', neutrophil leucocytosis or eosinophilia is seen. In late stages of the disease associated with marrow infiltration, pancytopenia and leucoerythroblastic anaemia occur.

Histopathology

Hopefully, diagnosis will be made in the early stages of the disease by biopsy of affected nodes. The histological appearances are pleomorphic, but the diagnosis of Hodgkin's disease cannot be made with certainty unless characteristic giant cells are seen (Reed–Sternberg cells).

Other histological features are of prognostic importance, e.g. the amount of lymphocytic infiltration into the tissue and the degree of fibrosis. Four histological types are generally recognised:

Lymphocyte predominant
Nodular sclerosing   Worsening
Mixed cellularity   prognosis
Lymphocyte depleted

Clinical Staging

Careful clinical and pathological staging is essential, since treatment differs between stages. The generally accepted clinical stages are:

Stage I   one lymph node group affected on one side of the diaphragm

Stage II   two affected lymph node groups on one side of the diaphragm

Stage III   nodal groups involved on both sides of the diaphragm, with or without splenic disease

Stage IV involvement of non-nodal tissues and organs, particularly liver and bone marrow.

Further subdivision of stages is made by adding suffixes A or B, indicating the presence or absence of systemic symptoms. Thus stage IIB may be associated with fever, weight-loss or sweating, all of which symptoms are absent in IIA disease.

In order to examine inaccessible lymphoid tissue, and therefore to make staging of the disease more accurate, it is usual to perform x-rays of the chest and abdomen, abdominal lymphangiography (with or without ultrasound or CT screening of the abdomen) and bone marrow biopsy. More advanced disease than was at first suspected may be found when the results of these investigations are reviewed. Unless late-stage disease has already been diagnosed, a staging laparotomy is performed, with biopsy of liver and para-aortic nodes, splenectomy, and raising of the ovaries to the midline lower abdominal wall, so that they may be shielded from subsequent radiotherapy.

Splenectomy serves several purposes. It represents biopsy of a potentially involved site and removal of diseased tissue. Any subsequent radiotherapy is also made easier, since radiotherapy to the spleen may injure the upper pole of the left kidney, and splenectomy renders the blood count more resistant to the effects of cytotoxic therapy.

Treatment

It is usual to employ radiotherapy for treatment of early stages of the disease (I and II), and chemotherapy for stage IV disease. Both modalities of treatment are employed in stage III disease.

Radiotherapy is usually given in wide fields to encompass all nodes on the involved side of the diaphragm. For disease above the diaphragm, a mantle field is employed. The term 'mantle' refers to the resemblance of the field to the shape of a gas mantle (Fig. 6.10). For disease below the diaphragm, an inverted Y is used.

First-choice chemotherapy in Hodgkin's disease is a combination of mustine, vincristine (Oncovin), procarbazine and prednisone (MOPP). Usually this regime is given in 14-day courses, repeated each month for 6–8 courses.

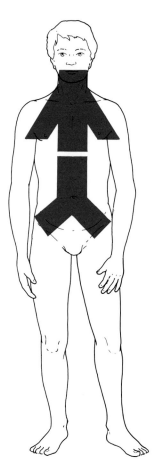

Fig. 6.10 *Mantle and inverted-Y radiation fields for treatment of Hodgkin's disease above and below the diaphragm.*

More than 50% of cases of Hodgkin's disease can be expected to be cured, or to die of other causes, when modern methods of staging and treatment are used.

NON-HODGKIN'S LYMPHOMAS

This group of disorders comprises neoplastic proliferations of the cellular components of lymphoid tissue. Unfortunately, ignorance of the pathological mechanisms involved has led to a plethora of histological classifications. These classifications are variously based on the structural characteristics of the nodes involved, the degree of differentiation of the cells involved, the morphology of these cells, and their immunological type.

The majority of non-Hodgkin's lymphomas arise from B cells of the lymph-node cortex (p. 17). Although older classifications recognised lymphocytic and histiocytic variants, the 'histiocyte' is in fact a large lymphocyte. True histiocytic lymphoma, involving cells of the monocyte–macrophage series, is very rare.

The histological feature most closely related to prognosis is the pattern of lymph-node involvement, either nodular or diffuse. As in Hodgkin's disease, nodular infiltration is associated with a better prognosis than is diffuse infiltration. Although many attempts at further classification have been made on the basis of the cytology of the malignant cells, the biological and prognostic value of such classifications remains controversial.

Clinical Features

As with Hodgkin's disease, a frequent presentation is with lymphadenopathy, which may be generalised or localised. In general, involvement of the lymphoid tissue of the gastrointestinal tract is commoner in non-Hodgkin's lymphomas than in Hodgkin's disease, and generalised disease at presentation is commoner in non-Hodgkin's lymphomas. While clinical staging is important in determining treatment, this does not usually include laparotomy. Systemic symptoms such as weight-loss, anorexia, malaise, sweating and fever become more apparent with generalised disease and are more prominent in high-grade (more malignant) types.

Blood Count

Spill-over of lymphoma cells into the blood may occur, resulting in a lymphocytosis. Usually the bone marrow is involved at this stage of the disease. When the lymphocytes are small and mature, the disease is indistinguishable from chronic lymphocytic leukaemia. Bone-marrow biopsy is an essential staging procedure in the investigation of non-Hodgkin's lymphoma.

Treatment

Localised disease is treated by radiotherapy, in similar fashion to Hodgkin's disease, while generalised disease requires chemotherapy. Chemotherapy with chlorambucil and prednisone may effectively control well-differentiated lymphocytic disease akin to CLL. Combination chemotherapy is required for more poorly differentiated diffuse disease. Cyclophosphamide, vincristine and prednisone (COP) is a frequently used combination. More powerful therapy for aggressive disease is provided by adding hydroxydaunorubicin (Adriamycin) to this regime (CHOP). Elderly patients tend to tolerate the more toxic schedules badly.

In such a pleomorphic group of disorders it is difficult to give accurate prognostic information. Nodular lymphomas may frequently be associated with survival times of 7–10 years but, in the diffuse varieties, 2–3 years is more usual.

RARE VARIANTS OF NON-HODGKIN'S LYMPHOMA

Because of their specific clinical or pathological features, certain non-Hodgkin's lymphoma variants have come to be regarded as specific entities.

Burkitt's Lymphoma

This is a tumour of B-cell type which particularly afflicts children in those areas of Equatorial Central Africa where malaria is endemic. A particularly common presentation is with massive tumours of the mandible and maxilla, but any organ of the body may be affected. There is little lymphadenopathy.

The Epstein–Barr virus (EBV) has been isolated from lymphoma cells, and it is postulated that, in persons exposed to malaria, this virus may cause Burkitt's lymphoma. In normal persons, the virus causes glandular fever (infectious mononucleosis). This lymphoma initially responds well to many cytotoxic agents, but is difficult to cure.

Waldenström's Disease

Like myeloma, this lymphoproliferative disorder is associated with diffuse bone marrow infiltration and secretion of paraprotein. However, the paraprotein is IgM in type (cf. IgG or IgA, most common in myeloma), and hypercalcaemia, bone pain and renal failure do not occur, while lymphadenopathy is often found. The cells infiltrating bone marrow, and sometimes present in the blood, show a characteristic morphological appearance halfway between plasma cells and lymphocytes.

This disorder responds to alkylating agents such as chlorambucil and cyclophosphamide.

Sézary's Syndrome

Infiltration of the skin with erythroderma is the prime feature of this T-cell neoplasm. There is a peripheral blood lymphocytosis, and many of the lymphocytes show a characteristic cleft nucleus.

Hairy-Cell Leukaemia

In this disorder, the spleen and bone marrow are heavily infiltrated with cells showing distinctive cytoplasmic projections (hairy cells), though lymph nodes are largely spared. Despite the name given to the disorder, blood involvement is variable. The disease often runs a chronic course and chemotherapy is usually not indicated.

Splenectomy may be beneficial when the spleen is substantially enlarged.

Further Reading

Chapter 1

Hoffbrand A.V., Lewis, S.M. (1981). *Postgraduate Haematology*, 2nd edn. London: William Heinemann Medical Books.

Roitt I.M. *Essential Immunology*, 4th edn. Oxford: Blackwell Scientific Publications.

Chapter 2

de Gruchy G.C.(1978). *Clinical Haematology in Medical Practice*, 4th edn. Oxford: Blackwell Scientific Publications.

Wintrobe M.M. (1981). *Clinical Haematology*, 8th edn. Philadelphia: Lea & Febiger.

Chapter 3

Cash J.D., ed (1976). Blood Transfusion and Blood Products. *Clinics in Haematology*; **5**: No. 1.

Clarke C.A. (1975). *Rhesus Haemolytic Disease – selected papers and abstracts with commentaries*. Lancaster: Medical and Technical Publishing Co. Ltd.

Conrad M.E., ed (1981). Transfusion Problems in Haematology. *Seminars in Haematology*; **17**: No. 2.

Mollison P.L. (1982). *Blood Transfusion in Clinical Medicine*, 9th edn. Oxford: Blackwell Scientific Publications.

Petz L.D., Swisher S.N. (1981). *Clinical Practice of Blood Transfusion*. Edinburgh: Churchill Livingstone.

Race R.R., Sanger R. (1975). *Blood Groups in Man*, 8th edn. Oxford: Blackwell Scientific Publications.

Slichter S.J. (1980). Controversies in Platelet Transfusion Therapy. *Annual Review of Medicine*; **31**: 509–540.

Zimmerman D.R. (1973). *Rh – The Intimate History of a Disease and its Conquest*. New York: Macmillan.

Chapter 4

Mustard J.F., Packham M.A. (1977). Normal and Abnormal Haemostasis. In *Haemostasis: British Medical Bulletin*; **33**: 187–191.

Forbes C.D., Prentice C.R.M. (1981). Physiology and Biochemistry of Blood Coagulation and Fibrinolysis. In *Disorders of Blood*, eds Hardisty R., Weatherall D.

Lowe G.D.O., Forbes C.D., eds (1982). *Unsolved Problems in Haemophilia*. M.T.P. Press.

Chapter 5

Bloom A.L., Thomas D.P., eds (1981). *Haemostasis and Thrombosis*. Edinburgh and London: Churchill Livingstone.

Chapter 6

Canellos G.P., ed (1979). The Lymphomas. *Clinics in Haematology*; **8**: No. 3.

Simone J.V., ed (1978). Acute Leukaemia. *Clinics in Haematology*; **7**: No. 2.

Videbaek A., ed (1975). Polycythaemia and Myelofibrosis. *Clinics in Haematology*; **4**: No. 2.

Index